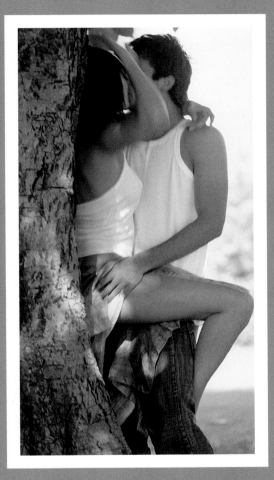

Quickies

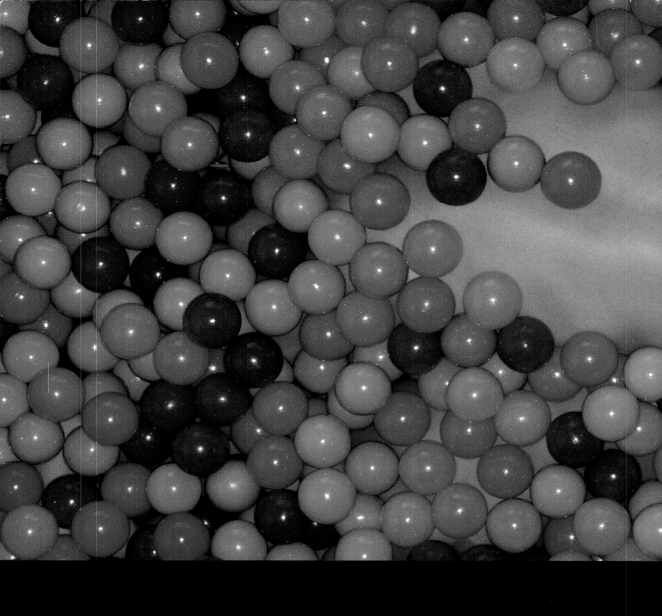

Must do it now! 62

When lust takes you unawares, take advantage by taking each other. Build the chance of spontaneous sex by keeping you both on sexual simmer with **foreplay that lasts forever**. Create the right environment for animal urges by **protecting your private time**.

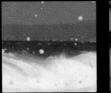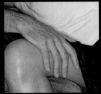
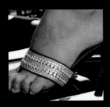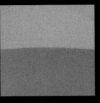
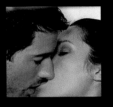

Three minutes to spare 86

Use them wisely. But who needs three minutes? You can have **sparky sex in 60 seconds**... There are plenty of **quick ways to climax** if you're prepared to **make a little time for making whoopee**.

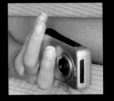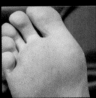
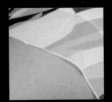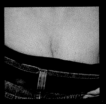

Just for kicks 100

Want to have **saucier, spicier sex**? Need to **entice your partner to try the kinky stuff**? If you're up for down-and-dirty sex, this is the chapter for you! Find out more about **naughty stuff and why you should try it**.

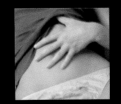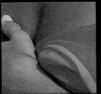

Use it or lose it

"Remember spontaneous sex? Impulsive, animalistic sex? Sex like it used to be in the beginning? Want to get all that back? Here's how..."

Apart from the odd, particularly perky pair, very few long-term couples clock up regular and riveting flesh-feasts. Lots of people complain about not having enough sex and there are two main reasons why they're not: zero time and low desire. "Busy" is today's buzzword and let's face it, after a four-hour dreadfully dreary meeting, a one-hour commute, dealing with kids

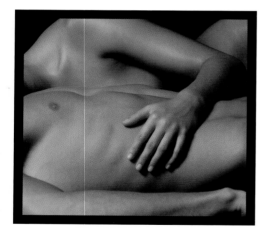

and/or routine chores, it's not surprising you're not removing each other's clothes with your teeth as the theme song of your favorite TV show beckons in the background. Problem is, even when we do have time for sex, it often still doesn't make it to the top of the I'll Die If I Don't Do It list. There's a good reason why. If you don't put the effort in, long-term sex is boring. Hell, short-term sex is boring if you don't mix things up a bit! *Quickies* aims to address these common problems by tackling things on two levels.

First, it delivers quick, fun sex ideas which you can find time for – some take a mere minute! Second, the ideas are fresh and quirky enough to make your sexual systems sit up and take notice. Public fondling, bold, bolshy out-there advances, the odd dip of toes in the kinky pool – it's all in here. And there's lots of less outrageous moves for the less confident and courageous. Original stuff (I hope, anyway!). While I've got nothing against the sexy-nightie-plus-candles-and-rosepetals-on-the-bed scenarios, your brains and your bits have probably been there, done that several (million) times already. It helps a little because at least you're making An Effort – but often making An Effort actually worsens the situation, rather than improving it. If you resort to clichés, you start to feel like one yourselves: sad sit-com characters rather than sexy beings, raring to go.

I've tried to make the suggestions in this book low-effort and time-efficient but also slightly risqué and a tad daring. So not only will you suddenly have time for sex, the excitement factor should soar upwards, toward if not immediately through the roof (and eventually way beyond that house extension which is currently taking all your attention). Let's come clean here (just don't make it a habit): if, when you do have sex, it's jesusthatwas*glorious* type of sex, chances are you'll make time for it. The way to keep your sex life skipping along nicely, rather than limping and dragging its feet, is to have lots of it and to make sure a good proportion is interesting and varied.

Let's come clean here: If, when you do have sex, it's jesusthatwas*glorious* type of sex, chances are you'll make time for it.

Although the whole point of quickies is "fast food sex", you should, when possible, mix in longer sessions. They don't have to be marathon, extreme-orgasm boot camp affairs where even the neighbours light up a cigarette when you're finally done and dusted. Just less time restricted, a little lazier, and with a heavy emphasis on soppy rather than sparky sex. The mid- to long-term effect of all this is interesting. Most couples find exploring new, previously uncharted territories boosts their appetite for sex. It's the equivalent of adding five fab gourmet meals to an if-it's-Monday-it-must-be-meatloaf food regime. Your taste buds can't help but be energized! The end result: you both want sex more often, and enjoy it more when you do.

Quickies is designed as an inspirational book, with bite-size, stand-alone pieces of advice and information. Open it at any page and you'll find a self-contained tip (or five). The photos are meant either to make you giggle or to get your juices flowing: use them as fantasy-fodder or as a spring-board for ideas. The suggested times accompanying some photographs aren't meant to be taken literally. They're designed to add atmosphere and plant wicked ideas in your head of when might be a good time, if you were to attempt what's pictured. Of course, you know and I know (and most importantly the police and your nosy, sex-starved, jealous neighbours know) that having sex outside in public view may be illegal. But then again, so is having anal sex in some parts of America and flashing an ankle in Saudi Arabia. It's all about being a bit sensible so check out the little "risk factor" hearts, do your sums (possible pleasure vs. possible embarrassment/arrest) and assess the situation. If you feel the risk is bordering on downright irresponsible, give it a miss until later. While we're on the subject of being sensible, please do take note that safe sex guidelines are not always given in this book because it is aimed at monogamous couples who have been tested and cleared for STDs and HIV. If this is not the case with you, always practice safe sex by using condoms and avoiding high-risk activities.

The sexy-nightie-plus-candles-and-rosepetals-on-the-bed scenarios tend to be overworked. If you resort to clichés, you start to feel like one yourselves rather than sexy beings, raring to go.

Right! That's more than enough sensible stuff – back to being naughty! And naughty I hope you will be, because that's what will help immeasurably to heat things up. Adding (calculated) risk and danger to your sex life gives it edginess. "Comfortable" is a lovely state to be in if you're relaxing in front of a fire; it's not so helpful for a racy sex session. Slightly uneasy sometimes works better.

Exploring new, previously uncharted territories boosts your appetite for sex. It's the equivalent of adding five fab gourmet meals to an if-it's-Monday-it-must-be-meatloaf food regime.

Quick sex works to rescue a sex life because it restores the elements which tend to fade when love kicks off the stilettos and pushes its feet into slippers. Remember the adrenaline rush? Impulsive, animalistic sex? Sex which provided a much-needed release without guilt and complications? Spontaneous sex? Sex with someone you saw as sexy, rather than a person who cooks the dinner or forgets to take the trash out? *Sex like it used to be in the beginning*. Wouldn't it be nice to get all that back?

Well now you can. Turn the page and start teasing.

Tracey X

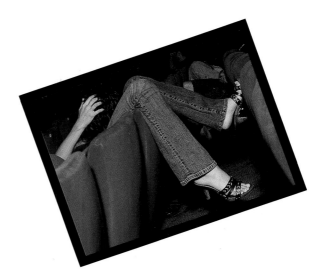

Always wanted to do it there!

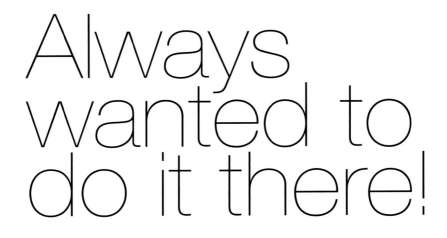

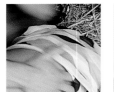 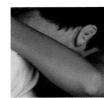 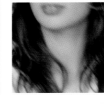 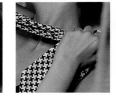

   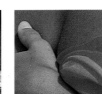 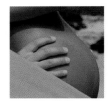

Certain locations and situations put a **fiendish twinkle** in everyone's eyes. Your parents' bed appealed as a teen because it was the ultimate no-go zone. **Work—the grown-up equivalent—is a top adult tempter**. Elevators and laundromats beckon because they offer tantalizingly brief periods of privacy. **And then there's the beach...**

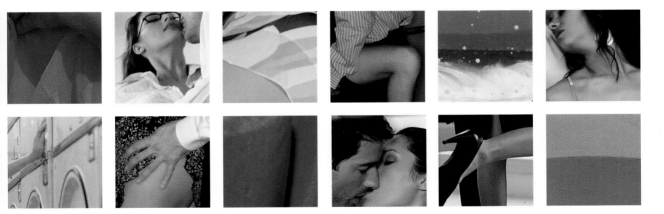

How to **get away with** sex in public

Not everyone will be as entranced at the sight of your partner's bare bottom pumping up and down as you are. Not being able to control your surroundings is all part of the thrill—but being arrested while cavorting in public isn't quite the kick we're after. Happily, this won't happen if you follow a few rules. It's fine to play on a plane under a blanket if there's no one sitting directly next to you, the cabin lights are off, and the man snoring across the aisle has his eye mask on. But getting it on in a public restroom when the line stretches from there to the bar isn't clever. In high-risk places, intercourse is out of the question. Instead, use the experience to be aroused rather than satisfied. Slip hands up and under shirts and tops, fondle genitals

In Japan, it's perfectly acceptable to strip naked and bathe together in public. Try kissing, though, and eyebrows are raised to the roof. In Western cultures, the opposite is true. No one cares if you touch tonsils, but a bared bod is sinful!

through clothing. Sucking fingers, dry humping, kissing—you can get away with them all, as long as you're quiet! The point of a quickie is fast, speedy release and instant gratification. Push clothes aside rather than remove; unbutton only when necessary and where possible; choose a position that you could unwind from in a flash if caught. Think about what you'll say if you do get caught: if it's a stranger, they'll probably be outta there before you can squeak "How embarrassing!". If they're frozen with shock, look sheepish and confess he just proposed and you got carried away/it's your anniversary and you vowed this is how you'd celebrate. And don't forget to zip up and tuck in after the deed is done and clean up after yourselves (sticky seats, condom wrappers, anything knocked over, etc.).

Boring textbooks, homework, and stern librarians telling us to shhhh! With memories like these, is it any wonder that as adults we have the urge to disrupt, disobey, and generally misbehave behind those conveniently high bookshelves?

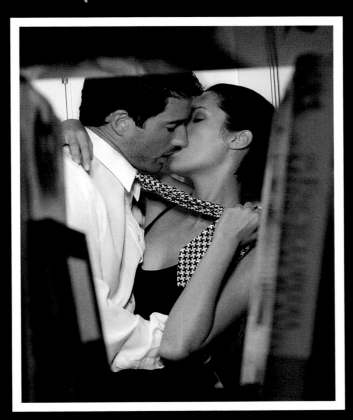

LIBRARY

lustylocation

oh!
oh!
oh!

orgasmoh!meter

♥♥♥
♥♥

riskfactor

1:45 pm

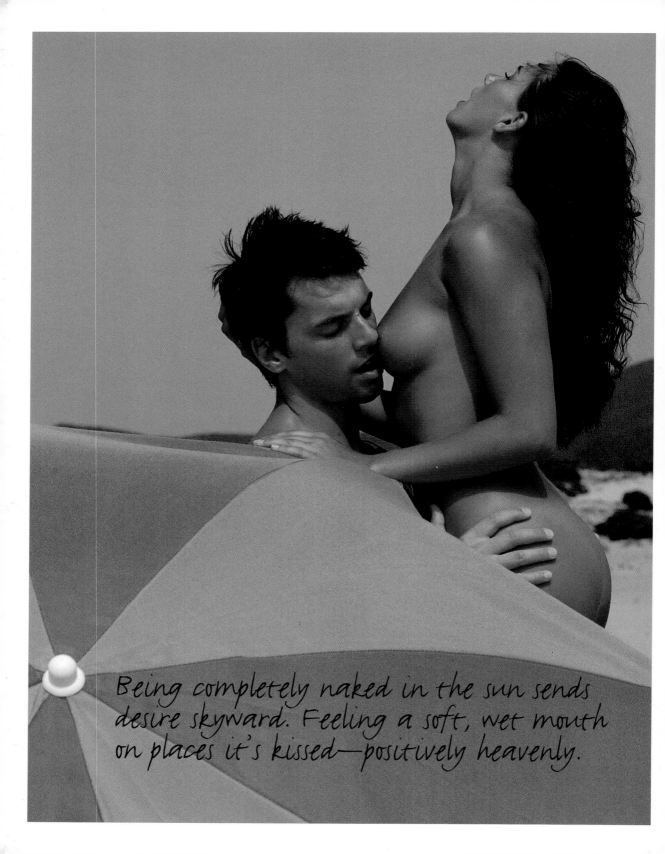

Being completely naked in the sun sends desire skyward. Feeling a soft, wet mouth on places it's kissed—positively heavenly.

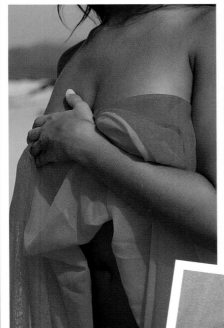

Sex in public requires nerve—and common sense. Setting up your beach umbrella next to a kid innocently building a sandcastle is asking for trouble. But a deserted, out-of-the-way beach is well worth the risk. Anxiety heightens desire. The problem with long-term love is that sex is too easy: it's available 24/7. Snuggled up spooning in your beds, sex is but a whispered invitation or a hopeful hand on a thigh away. Convenient, yes, but not terribly exciting. You're not supposed to have sex outside, and this is exactly why it amplifies every touch, making it seem a dozen times sweeter than it would indoors.

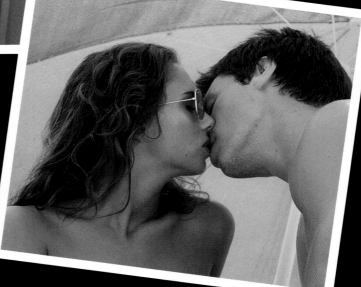

BEACH PARASOL

lustylocation

oh!
oh!
oh!

orgasmoh!meter

riskfactor

9:33 am

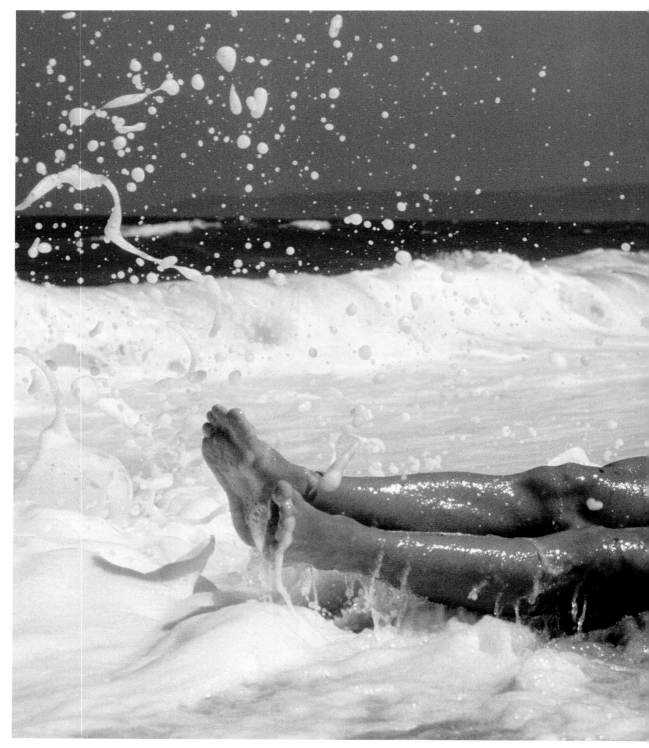

Wet inside and out, slippery limbs, crashing waves and inner

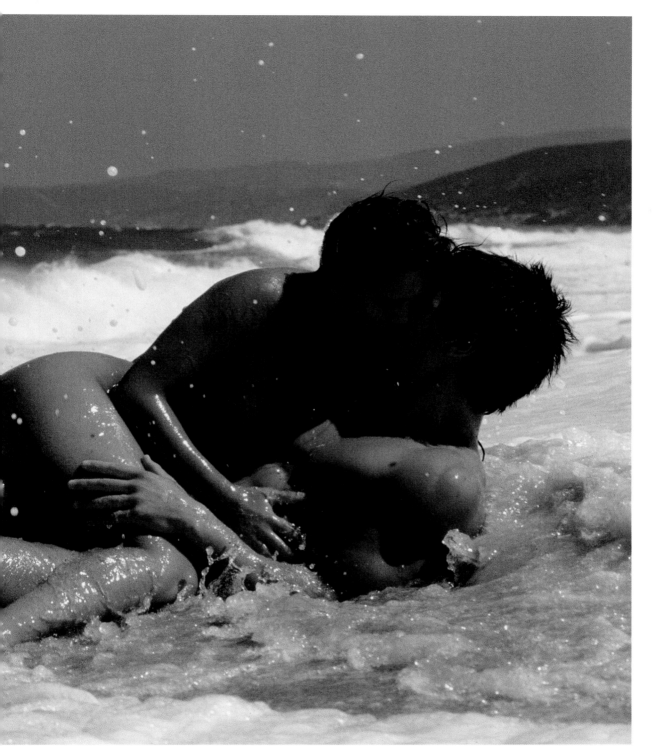

whirlpools—sea sex is both animal and dramatically romantic.

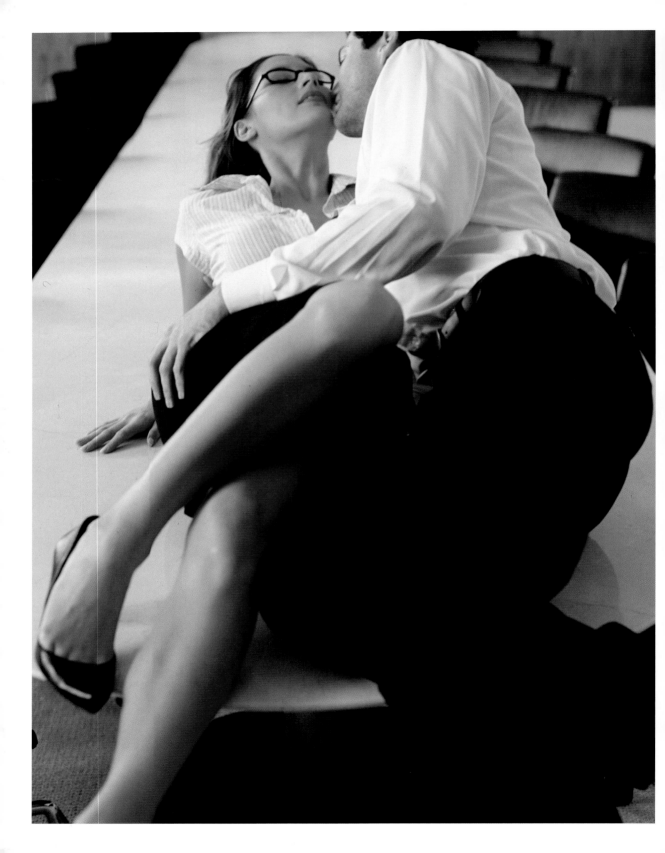

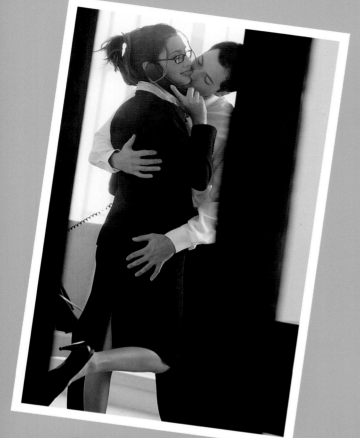

The office is a veritable hotbed of unrequited lust—the average meeting produces more in the way of creative sex fantasies about colleagues than business ideas! If you're lucky enough to be dating a workmate, the office has never been more fun—and photocopying never taken quite so long. But even if you're not, visiting a partner at work, when all but the cleaning staff have left, means you can recreate an office affair via roleplay. Pretend you've been longing to touch each other for months. Affair sex is addictive because it's frowned upon and time-limited: anticipation and mounting desire make us frantic for satisfaction. Sex in a forbidden scenario, like on a boardroom table, has the same elements: you're half-excited, half-worried all day—will you get away with it? (Of course you will!)

BOARDROOM

lustylocation

oh!
oh!
oh!

orgasmoh!**meter**

riskfactor

Stolen moments make us savor every last second. There's no time to be lazy, so full focus is given to sex.

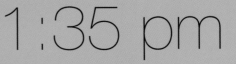

1:35 pm

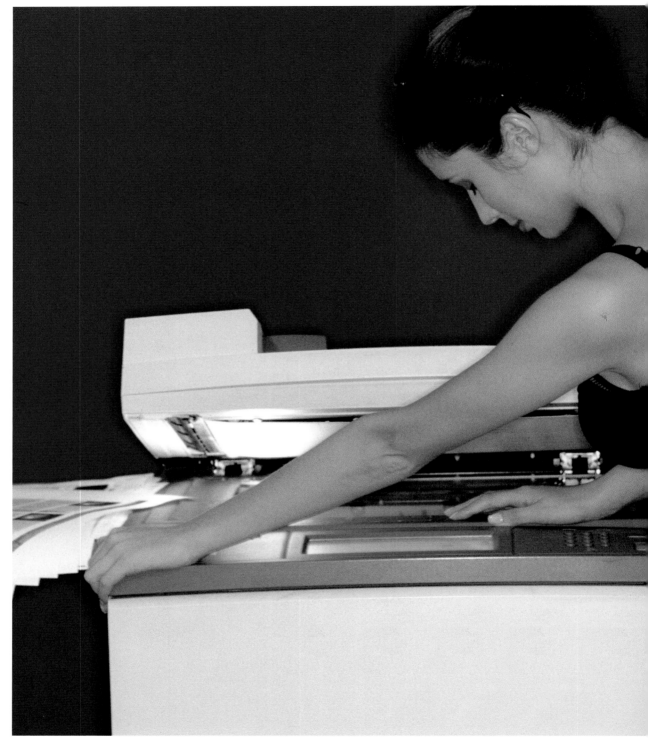

Office sex is super-risky and adrenalin-pumping. Exposed and

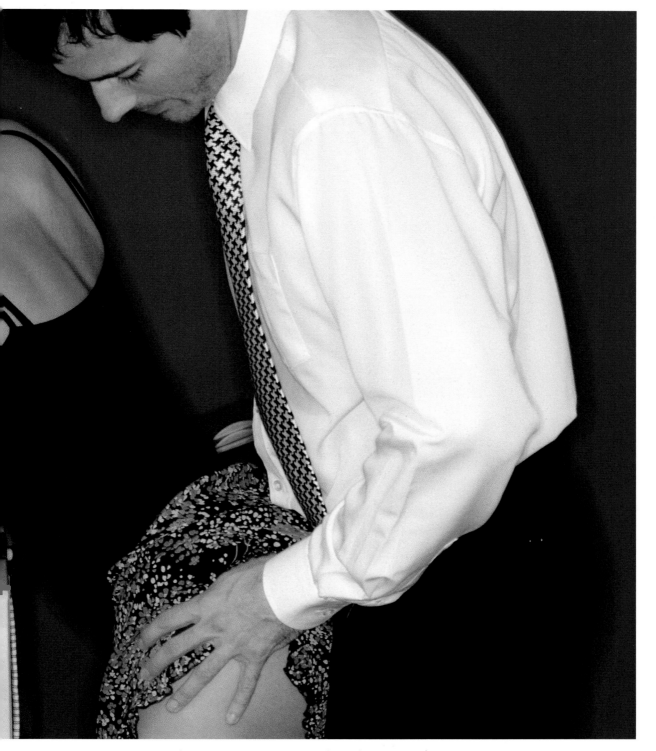

excited, a simple hand on your thigh can be electrifyingly erotic.

quick sex: the rules

1

accept responsibility for feeling sexy

The bed partner of the myth that says good sex "just happens" with zero effort from either of you is the one that says the rampant desire that had you shagging in closets at the beginning of your relationship will continue to tap you on the shoulder six months, sixteen months, and six years in. It won't. Sad but true, we lose desire for something once we've got it on tap. But it's also a myth that you can't get back what you once had. Research shows that people who have high libidos think about sex far more often than those with low desire, and that you can teach yourself to be more sexual—and to want sex with your partner more often. Train your brain to turn yourself on every day, in every situation. A shower is far more sense-ational if you use scented gels, soaping yourself the way a lover would. On the morning and evening commutes, find something you find attractive about everyone on the bus or train (with discreet and stolen glances rather than obvious stares!). When you're talking to a colleague, focus on their hands and remember what your partner did with theirs last time you had great sex. Savor tastes on your tongue, dress in clothes you know you look good in, read erotic books, hang sexy pictures in your bedroom, rent X-rated movies... The more you start thinking about sex, the more you keep thinking about sex. It's not your lover's job to keep you turned on, it's yours.

2

use a lubricant

Most men can get an erection in the time it takes her to say "Wanna do it?". Women's arousal systems are, sadly, a tad slower. During relaxed lovemaking, there's time for the vagina to lubricate and expand: during quick sex, you both need to be ready for immediate action. Adding lubricant speeds up the female arousal process by instantly providing what her body usually takes a little while to provide naturally. With gentle but slippery hands, you can dive straight for her good bits, guaranteeing pleasure, not pain. Lubricant also artificially prepares her for quick penetration. Combine this with immediate, expert stimulation and you can shock her sexual system from "Whoa" to "Go" in under a minute. Leave tubes of lubricant in secret hiding places (the side of the sofa, the bathroom, the glove compartment of the car, in the office). You can also buy little sachets of travel-size lubricant to carry with you, for whenever and wherever.

3

mix quickies with longer sex

Fast, frenzied sex will do many nice things for your relationship: it reminds you both how much you like each other on a purely physical basis, it's unplanned, impulsive sex that keeps the "Aren't we naughty?" buzz alive, and there is no argument against the fact that quick sex, rather than no sex, keeps you connected as a couple. One survey shows that couples who have lots of quickies kiss, cuddle, and hold hands more than those who have less frequent, longer sessions. Having sex in unusual places adds the danger and urgency that is often missing from long-term sex, and doing it in places other than the bed forces you to try new positions and means of stimulation you wouldn't normally bother with (most of us are lazy buggers, really). But if all you're having is quick sex, you're completely missing the point.

A good sex life is balanced, and you need a variety of sex sessions to nurture all parts of your emotional and sexual selves. Lusty and loving. Long and short. It's totally acceptable to have quick sex eight out of ten times you make love. But when you do have time, make the effort. A sensible two-week mix for busy couples is to include four to six low-effort, minutes-long turn-ons (you'll find ideas for these scattered throughout the book), at least four quickies (anywhere from five minutes to fifteen), and at least one session that lasts up to an hour (or more). In total, that's around an hour and a half every two weeks. Considering most of us spend around two hours per night parked in front of the TV, that's a pretty effective use of time, wouldn't you say?

4

stop thinking sex = intercourse

Rethink what you mean by "sex." A quickie means quick sex of any kind, not necessarily intercourse. Think of "sex" as anything that makes you feel sexy—teased as well as totally sated. Two minutes of oral sex is just long enough to get everything standing to attention… and wanting more, more, more when that mouth is taken away. Teasing each other physically—arousing your sexual systems, then leaving them to simmer—whets the appetite and encourages anticipatory sex. Spontaneity, often lost long-term, gets replaced by something far more delicious: knowing what's coming and exactly how they're going to do it. A deliciously sexy, long, smooch and neck kissing, a hot text from your lover that makes you instantly wet—all these things count as "sex" sessions.

Learn to enjoy parts of sex and parts of your bodies, rather than always devouring the whole thing. Impose rules to introduce limitations designed to get you both begging for more: hands only, tongues only, penetration only, breasts only, genitals only, only she's allowed to touch, only he's allowed to touch. Then stop—part company for a while if you have to—and enjoy the hot rush of desire you feel from your encounter.

quick sex: the rules

5 — seize the moment—and don't stress

Give up on only having sex when everything is perfect for it. Wait until you're both looking fab and feeling horny, have your best underwear on, you've got time, the kids aren't home, you've got hours to spare and all the energy in the world, and you've got about as much chance of having regular sex as I have waking up looking like Angelina Jolie. Real life rarely affords the perfect circumstances for sex, so you have to take it when and where you can. Give into spontaneous animal passion and let lust take care of all the niceties. Quick sex isn't about comfort, candles, and flattering lighting: it's raw, intense and rough-and-ready. You can't undress in "could-get-caught" locations; besides, there's an animal passion to being hastily half-dressed. Panties roughly pulled to one side, jeans around your ankles—it's reminiscent of those heady, adolescent fumblings… Who cares if the dinner gets burned, you're five minutes late to the office, neither of you has showered, or the kids watched garbage TV for ten minutes longer than you'd have liked. Sometimes an over-organized sex session guarantees you a bland, orchestrated one. You both feel like you're in some corny romantic movie, and the pressure's on to get all Hollywood: worrying far too much about how it's looking on the outside, rather than focusing on what's happening on the inside. Much better to have a quick, passing grope that makes your blood surge for a few seconds and then leaves you glowing afterward.

6 — don't be orgasm-focused

The more quick sex encounters you have, the higher your libido will soar. The more orgasms you have, the more easily orgasmic you will become. Orgasms help develop strong nerve pathways to the source of stimulation in the brain. The better-traveled those pathways are, the higher your orgasmic potential, so the more you orgasm, the more easily you'll have them. But to expect an orgasm every time you touch or arouse each other is both unrealistic and restrictive. The idea is to keep both of you permanently on sexual simmer: and that means anything from warming up to boiling over. You will have more orgasms by having lots of quick sex, but just because neither of you climaxed, it doesn't mean it didn't rate as a hot, sheet-clutching experience. Having said that, by all means up the odds of one by shamelessly pressing all your partner's known triggers, and up her chances by choosing clitoris-friendly positions. Ensuring that you or she can stimulate her during penetration helps immeasurably; so does putting her on top or having rear-entry sex. Both positions guarantee you're hitting her front vaginal wall, which appears to be responsible for women having "no hands" vaginal orgasms.

7

learn from affair sex

There's a reason why people stray—and it's a good one. (Why else would they risk losing their lover, kids, and very often a life they're quite contented with most of the time?) Affairs don't just provide sex, they provide a particular type of sex: exciting sex. Long-term couples have cuddly sex, familiar sex, damn satisfying sex—but the adjective that disappears the most rapidly is "exciting." Familiarity makes you shy (it's harder to say "While you're down there, put this in your mouth" to your wife, on her knees picking up the kids' toys, than it was when she was your wicked girlfriend), and regularity effectively robs you both of mystery. But there are lots of qualities of affair sex that you can emulate in your relationship.

The intensity in affairs is often caused by time limitations: enforce your own deadlines on sex sessions and you'll achieve a similar effect. When affairees text, email, or call, the theme of each communication is lust and longing. Long-term lovers use electronics for mundane purposes ("Pick up some milk on your way home, honey"). Rediscover technology as the sexy stimulator it can be. Recreate the affair sensation of savoring every last, precious second by making dates to see each other outside the home. Coffee at lunchtime when you both have to get back to work makes us listen more and engage with our partners far more than when chatting at home. Affair sex is rarely done in the home environment—and that's why it feels great. Sex on vacations or in a hotel is nearly always better than sex at home, so find plenty of excuses to be Mr. & Mrs. Jones.

8

choose your time

People complain a lot about mismatched libidos: one wanting more sex than the other. But often it's a case of bad timing. Some people like nothing more than to be woken by a hopeful prod in the back and/or a tongue snaking its way up their thigh. Others would cheerfully cut off the tongue and any other offending appendages for an extra five minutes of shut-eye. If you're having a desire dysfunction, both keep a chart of when you feel like sex the most, then compromise from there. If you're a night person and he's a morning, a little afternoon delight could solve your problems. Take advantage of our natural biological highs. Our testosterone levels are highest when we first wake up, so it can be worth waking up a bit earlier. The most popular high desire day for women is just before ovulation—around 14 days after your period. When it comes to orgasms, men appear relatively unaffected month to month, but women are more likely to orgasm just before or during their period, because increased blood flow adds pressure to the pelvic area and there are high levels of progesterone. You might feel as though the record (a 43-second-long mega-orgasm for one very lucky woman, according to Masters and Johnson) is out of reach, but there's no need to be jealous of his orgasmic regularity. Women climax harder, longer, and more often in one session than men do.

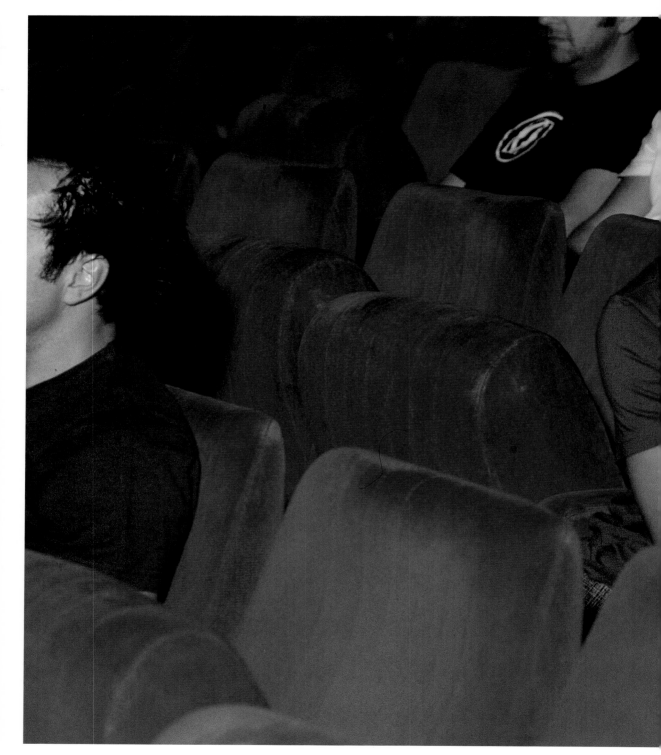

The movies take us back to our teens, when sex was forbidden,

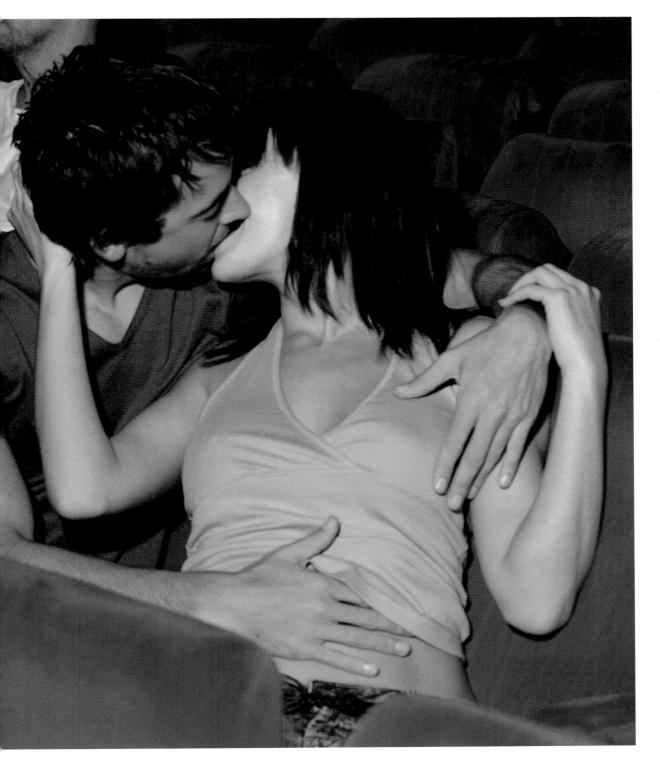

carnal crushes intense, and intimate touches constantly craved.

With time on your hands, why not make the most of his? All those sexy, squishing, swirling sounds... who could resist getting steamy?

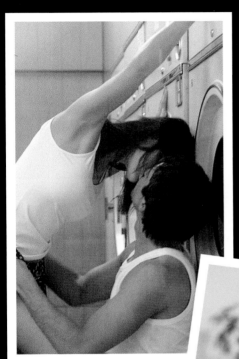

It's fast, opportunistic sex—and it beats the hell out of mindlessly watching your jeans and socks go around and around. A long skirt with nothing underneath is the perfect ready-whenever quick-sex outfit: it looks innocent, so you can be anything but. You stand to allow him easy access and to keep an eye on passing traffic or potential customers. Or try sitting with his back to the door, obscuring you, while you keep watch. It's a tad too risky to attempt penetration in such a public place, but a swift but discreetly delivered hand-job is achievable—and oh so appreciated.

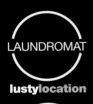

LAUNDROMAT

lustylocation

oh!
oh!
oh!

orgasm**oh!**meter

riskfactor

3:40 pm

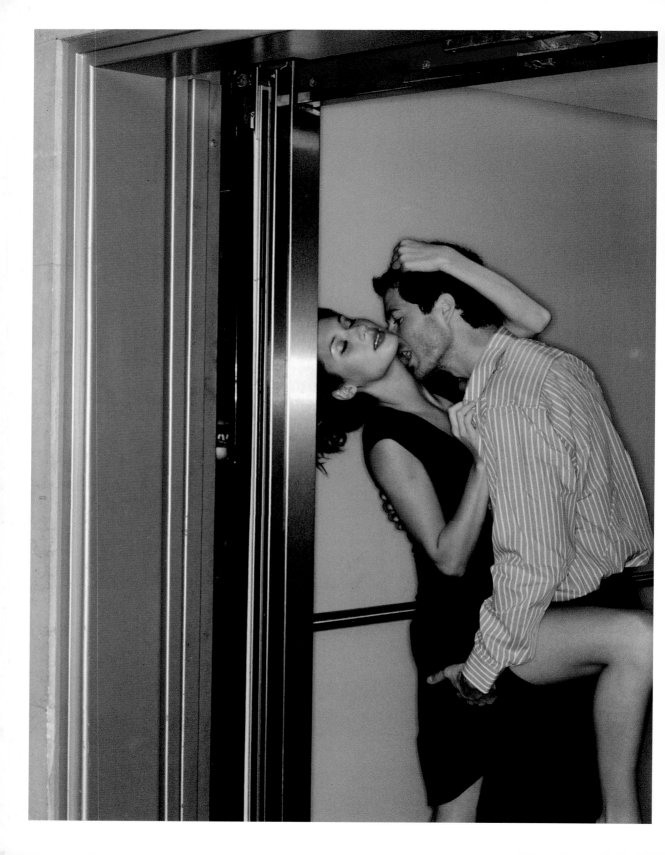

Having sex in an elevator (and actually getting away with it) requires nerves of steel and cunning planning. You don't have time to peel off lots of layers, so awkward-to-undo belts, too-tight, buttoned-up jeans, and lace-up shoes are all out. Instead, opt for loose pants with zippers, flared skirts you can lift up, baggy shirts you can easily get your hands under, and kick-off shoes. You need the naughtiness of being semi-naked but be able to look remotely composed (albeit not impeccably groomed) in the time it takes the door to slide open. Choose a standing-up position (this will be easier to extricate yourselves from), which allows one of you to keep your thumb firmly on the "doors closed" button. Keep hands and limbs away from the one labeled "emergency." Drape an item of clothing over the security camera and you should have at least three to five minutes before someone comes knocking. Assume panicked expressions if the door opens to reveal a security guard. You were locked in there! Thank God he rescued you! (Tee hee.)

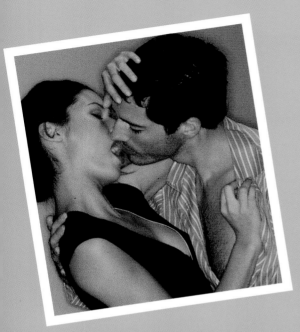

ELEVATOR

lustylocation

oh!
oh!
oh!

orgasmoh!meter

riskfactor

Doing it in an elevator tops most people's "Would Kill To Do It There" lust list. Going down, sir? And where would madam like me to take her?

6:37 pm

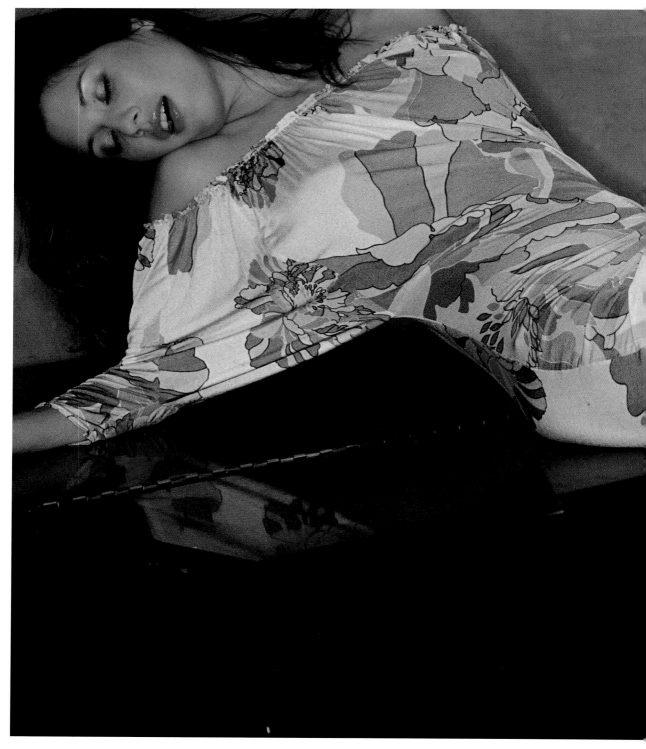

some movie scenes beg to be recreated. Make like Pretty

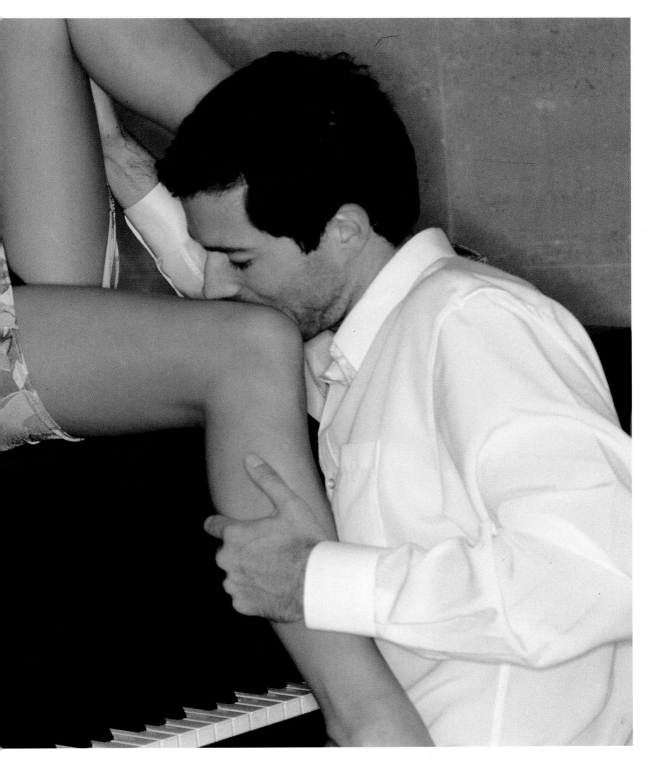

...woman and tinker with more than just the piano keys.

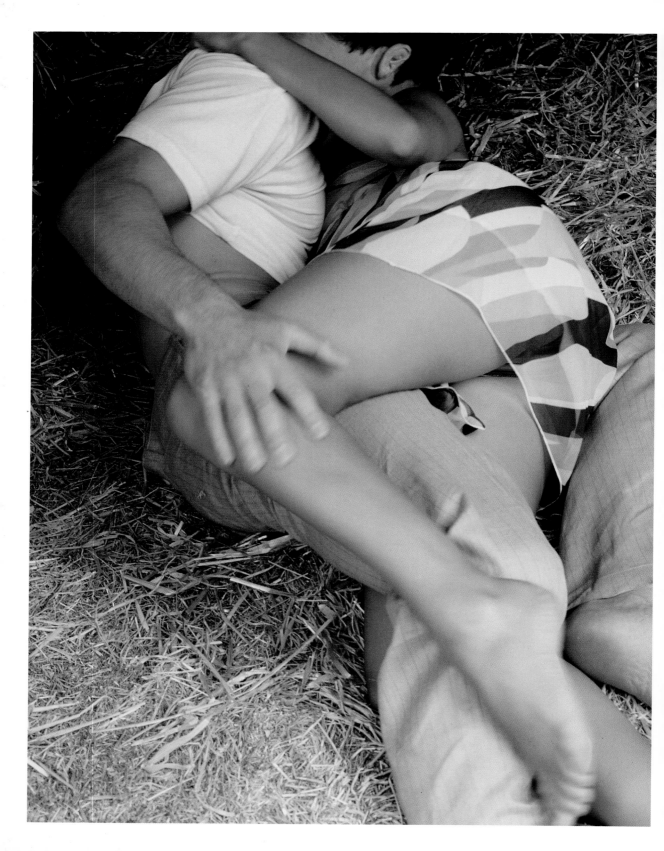

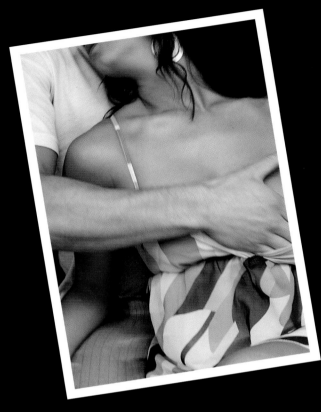

The joy of quick sex is not having to think about long-term comfort—which means you're far more likely to do it somewhere risqué or try a position that looks physically challenging. But here's a location that offers up a raunchy risk factor and a place to cuddle up after satisfying those carnal cravings. A barn is also a shelter from the sun or a cozy haven from dripping skies. And that's not the only thing that will be wet when you suggest the idea to her. Plenty of teenage girls are horse-crazy, spending their summers hanging around riding stables. Except most find they're spending more time eyeing up the shirtless, sexy guy cleaning out the stalls than the ponies in them. Take her back to those hormone-driven, confusingly consuming fantasies by role-playing a lusty stable-hand seducing an innocent.

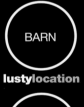

BARN

lustylocation

oh!
oh!
oh!

orgasmoh!meter

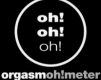

riskfactor

Get supersexy outdoors – without getting arrested! The sensation of straw on bare flesh and the smell of nature stir animalistic urges.

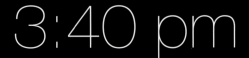

3:40 pm

Fun quickies

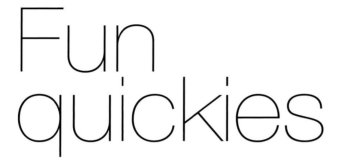

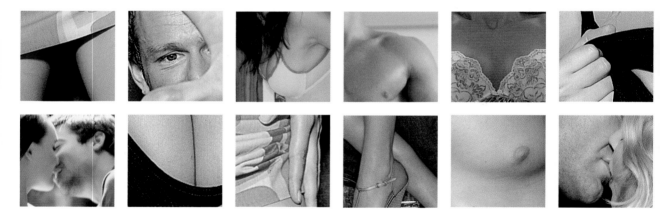

Having seriously good sex is one thing, having only serious sex quite another. **Playing games**, doing it with your socks still on, **laughing so hard** you can't even kiss—**sex is supposed to be fun**, remember? The more you play, **the longer both of you will stay**.

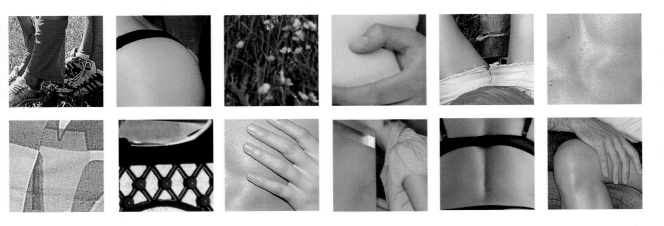

Frisky **fresh air frolics**

Pack a picnic, a sense of humor, and a playful attitude, and you're well on your way to a fun, sexy day out—not to mention a lasting, satisfying relationship. Taking sex out of your cozy, confined bedroom into the unpredictable great outdoors adds variety and excitement. Outdoor sex and the threat of discovery forces you to adopt new sex "rules." You're more likely to try a new position that looks erotic but uncomfortable because you're only in it for a minute or two! It also makes us break out of the restrictive "your turn, my turn" model. Most of us are brainwashed into thinking each sex session has to be a reciprocal one: you should both be doing things to each other at the same time and should repay a sexual favor the

Country quickies bring you back down to earth— literally. All that playful romping works up a sweat, releasing your natural scent, which is packed with potent chemical attractants. Nature's aphrodisiac!

minute yours is over. This is all very PC, but your attention is always split. Also, just as a massage never feels quite so good when you know you have to give one back immediately afterward, neither does "you then me" sex! Quick sex doesn't allow the must-give-and-take principle to operate because there's no time. Instead, sex becomes "your turn this time, my turn next time"—a far more pleasurable split, don't you think? It also means you're in charge of your own orgasms. It's generally harder for women to climax quickly, but you can up the chances. Grind in a circular motion as he thrusts, and push your pubic bone against him to stimulate the clitoris. Clench your vaginal muscles, buttocks, and upper thigh muscles to increase blood flow (and therefore sensation) to the pelvic area. Get him to press down on your lower abdomen to massage the inner clitoris (what you see is just the tip) and remember to breathe as you orgasm—it makes it more intense.

Playing together is as essential to good sex as orgasm is. A one-minute belly-laugh can relax you for up to 45 minutes afterward! Laugh more and you'll love more.

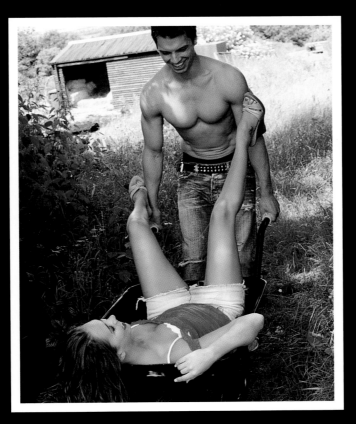

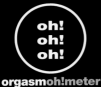

FARM

lustylocation

oh!
oh!
oh!

orgasm**oh!**meter

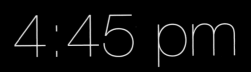

riskfactor

4:45 pm

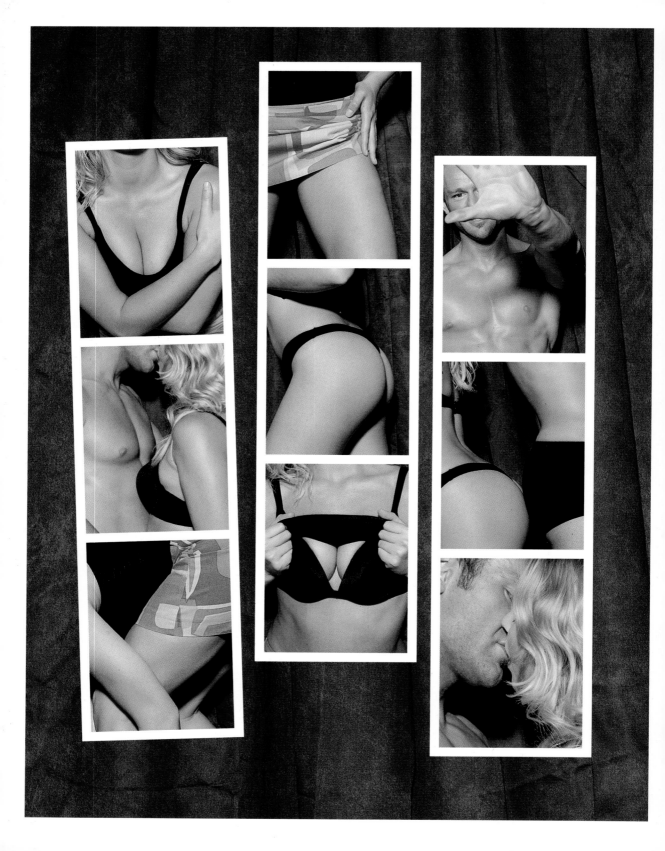

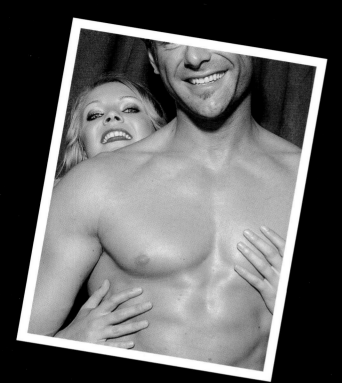

Photographic evidence of an adventurous sex life is not always a good thing. Fuming exes have a habit of recycling racy Polaroids, sticking them under your new partner's windshield wiper or leaving them in their mailbox. But if you've been together a while and there's a high trust factor, cavorting in front of a camera works well. Doing naughty things in a public photo booth is good (un)clean fun (the very best kind). Pics pinned on your bedroom mirror act as a permanent reminder of how sexy and attractive you both are and—most importantly—how well you play together. When you stomp into the bedroom and slam the door after arguing over something trivial, your eyes glance over to see the two of you laughing and… perspective is restored!

PHOTO BOOTH

lustylocation

oh!
oh!
oh!

orgasmoh!**meter**

Playing in a public photo booth, the unabashed strip down to their underwear; the shy settle for a long, sexy kiss.

riskfactor

4:50 pm

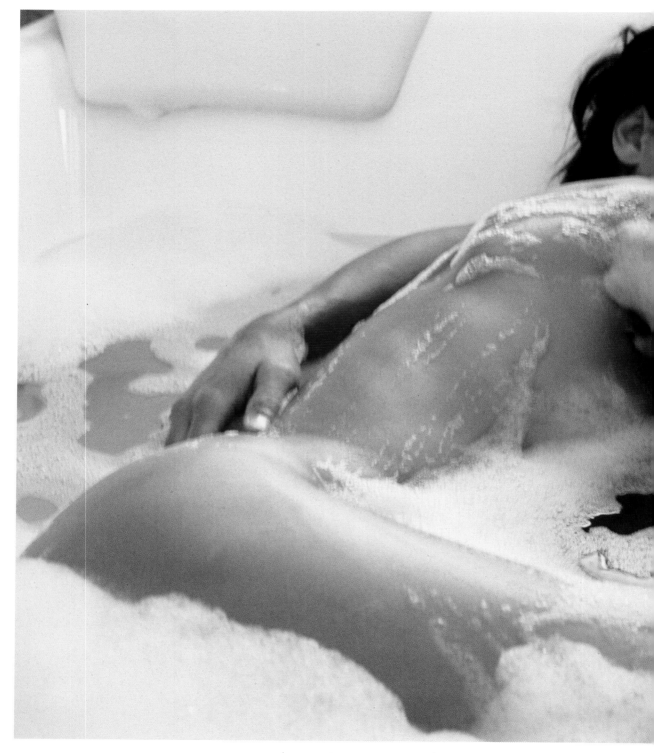

We associate Jacuzzis with opulence and luxury. Not surprising,

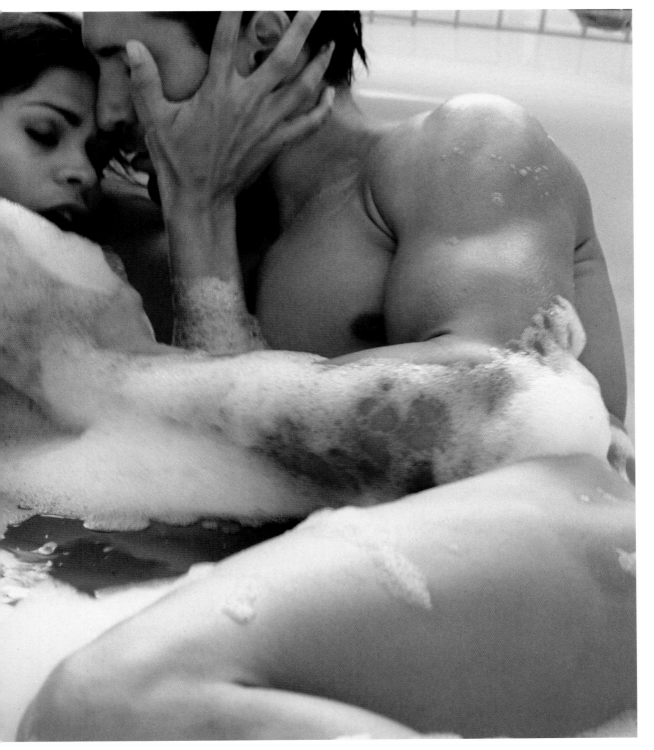

then, that it's the ultimate hedonistic sex fantasy for many.

Running raises your heart rate—
but so do other things! Time out
for another kind of knee-trembler.

11:45 am

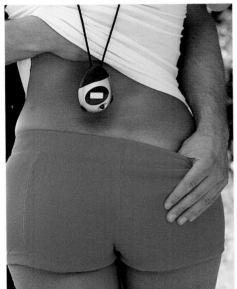

Standing positions are better for high-risk situations for an obvious reason—you can extricate yourselves easily and make a run for it! You stand with your back to him, bend over, and put your palms on your ankles, the floor or a convenient level rock or fence. He pulls your running shorts down, quickly unzips, applies some (prepacked) lubricant, then penetrates, holding your waist for balance. This position handily elevates your buttocks, angling him straight for the nerve-packed God-that-feels-good front vaginal wall.

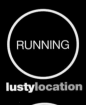

lustylocation

RUNNING

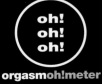

oh!
oh!
oh!

orgasm**oh!**meter

risk**factor**

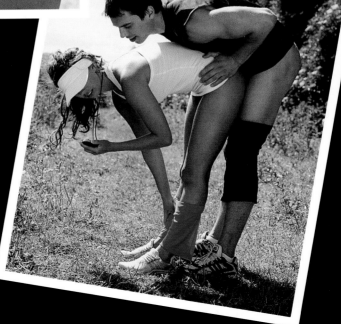

quickie essentials

1

❤ **A cheap, two-person tent**—it triples the outdoor possibilities, and with the flap open, you're not losing the feel.

❤ **A blanket**—protection for those bottoms, knees, and other vulnerable parts from hard, scratchy, or wet surfaces.

❤ **A waterproof mini vibrator**—for bringing her to orgasm in public places. If you're not within earshot of others, you can get away with murder.

❤ **Travel lube**—buy handy travel-size sachets or tubes. Make sure it's water- or silicone-based—less irritating and more staying power!

❤ **Sunscreen**—you'd be amazed at the tan marks produced by just 10 minutes with panties around your ankles.

❤ **Insect repellent and anti-itch cream**— waving your hands around to deflect pesky flies or mosquitoes dilutes the sexiness. So does madly scratching till you bleed.

❤ **Compact mirror**—to check the damage the quickie's done to your hair. Bits sticking up and pieces of twigs sticking out is what usually gives people away.

❤ **A credit card/cash**—to pay for a cab in case you have to get out of there fast.

❤ **A drink**—not only do you get a headache from dehydration, no saliva means dry kisses and dreadful oral sex.

2

indoor treats you'll have lying around

❤ **Sexy books and movies**—it doesn't have to be porn, just whatever each of you finds erotically arousing to read, read to each other, watch, or have playing in the background.

❤ **Old pairs of tights, his old ties**—great for tying hands behind your back, tying each other to beds/chairs/whatever.

❤ **Toothpaste, ice-cubes, fizzy drinks**—put some in your mouth before dispensing oral for a terrific tingly sensation.

❤ **Razor**—to shave each other's pubes.

❤ **Eyemasks from the plane**—these make great blindfolds.

❤ **A selection of great underwear**—glam and gorgeous, suitably sleazy, something for "fat days."

❤ **Girlie mags**—to cheat during phone sex by reading out the good parts. Also a great masturbation aid.

❤ **A freestanding full-length mirror**—the simplest, most useful sex tool of all. Watch yourself, your partner, or both of you. (One way to find out what your orgasm face really looks like.)

3

❤ **A paddle or "soft" whip for spanking**—essential as props for any sort of power roleplay (and aren't they all about power?). Both look the part but won't leave a mark (unless you want them to, that is!).

❤ **A vibrator**—think about whether you want clitoral or vaginal stimulation, or both, and test it out for noise level and strength of vibration before you buy. Use together or solo to keep your sex drive revved.

❤ **A travel vibe**—consider an ultra-quiet fingertip micro vibrator. All you or he need to do is slip it on, position your finger, then hold it still. With no arm movement, there's little risk of getting caught.

❤ **Vibrating penis ring**—he attaches a tiny, battery-powered vibrator to his penis via an elastic band. If he grinds instead of thrusts, it gives her the best of both worlds.

AVOID anything expensive you think you'd get sick of—apart from vibrators and most of the above, the main buzz from a sex toy is novelty. Plenty of couples have had their fill (ahem) after one or two sessions. Set budgets for obvious gimmick toys and have realistic expectations—most toys actually don't do what they say on the box. But they are fun and terrific for breaking you out of a ritual rut and getting you laughing in bed!

4

It makes sense to pack a few sexual props and toys for that (hopefully) filthy weekend away, but if you don't feel like showing the nice man at the security checkpoint how they work, pay attention.

❤ **Where are you going?** If it's somewhere that has its own "red-light" district, it could be easier to buy a cheap version just to last the weekend you're there.

❤ **Pack obvious toys** in your suitcase, not your carry-on, and where possible, use micro- or travel-size versions to save space.

❤ **Pack innocent-looking scarves** and stockings for tie-up games and to use as blindfolds.

❤ **Consider the circumstances**. If you're traveling with friends or kids, you'll need ultra-quiet or noiseless toys. You might also consider investing in some "disguised" sex toys. Vibrators come disguised as lipsticks, objets d'art, pens, rubber ducks, dolphins, and cell phones. That savvy friend may raise her eyebrows on picking one up, but your grandma or two-year-old won't have a clue.

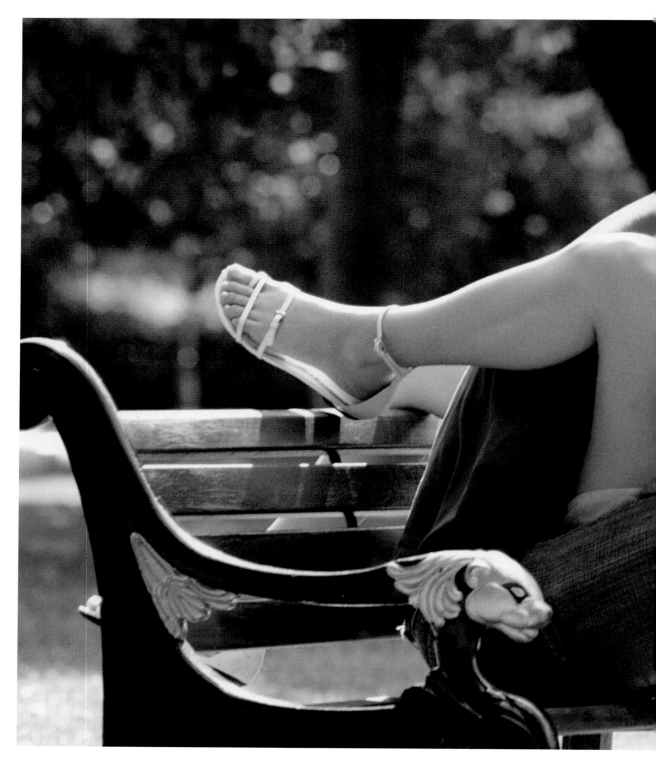

Having scoped out your rendezvous for interruptions and

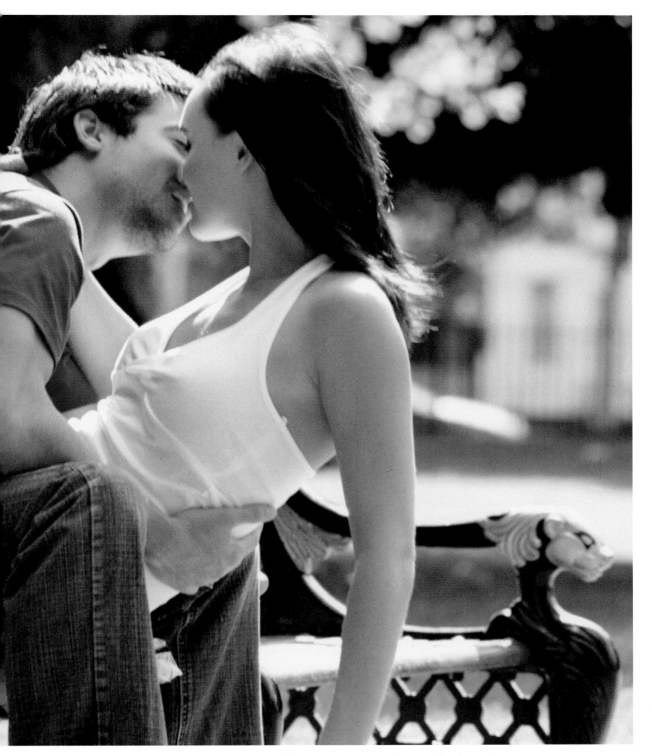

escape routes, you play in full view of the whole sky.

Have more, **want more**

Want more romance in your life? Well, have more sex! Sometimes those planned romantic dinners aren't what the sex therapist ordered. Facing each other across a restaurant table, surrounded by loved-up, just-got-out-of-bed-and-about-to-dive-straight-back-in-there couples can make you feel even more acutely aware you haven't "done it" in ages. If you're feeling estranged through lack of sex or affection, have a ten-minute quickie before you go out on your "date." And make it a sexy late-night bar rather than a stuffy restaurant. Even better if you spent the day before dispensing a few seconds-long sexual treats. You're feeling naughty having just been wanton, you're giggling instead of forcing smiles—and who cares if you

Couples who have regular sex get along better out of bed too: they communicate more effectively, show more affection, and have more energy. Couples who don't get enough sex argue more often and are irritable, angry, or depressed (sound familiar?).

have so many cocktails you want to spoon, not shag, when you get home. There's always tomorrow (wake-up sex, shower sex, sex before Sunday lunch with your parents).

Here's the thing: even if your desire level is so low you'd rather volunteer to do his tax return than wrap your mouth around his penis, all is not lost. US studies show a direct link between having sex and a high libido. Intercourse raises hormonal levels, which increase the brain chemicals associated with desire. Force yourself to have a few quickies and watch something rather amazing happen. Dread at "having" to have sex turns into anticipation. You might not feel like frequent sex, but your body sure as hell does! Sex is one of your body's greatest pleasure sources. Feed it a few bite-size portions and it becomes hungry for more.

d cool cocktail bar, flirt and
le home for more fun. Check
into an X-rated chatroom as
– outrageously lewd things to

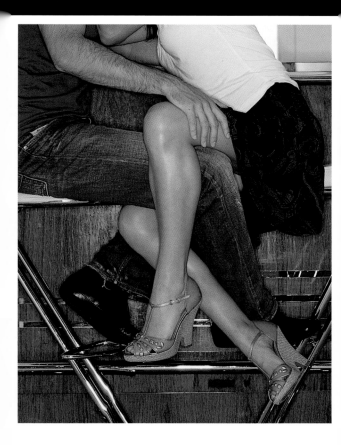

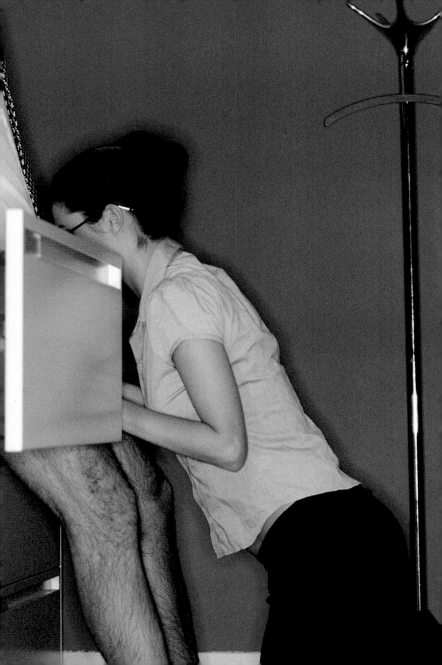

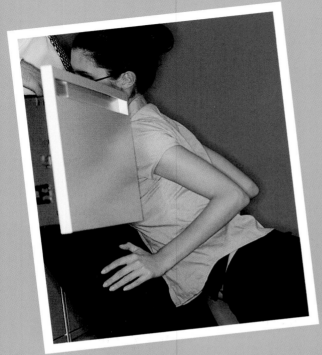

Something happens to us when we're left alone in a place that is normally packed with people. We're consumed by naughty urges to sneak a peek in the boss's top drawer, deliberately mess up that impeccably organized pen collection on a co-worker's desk—or do something else on it when our lover arrives to take us home. Greet him with an overly enthusiastic kiss hello and he won't take long to get the message.

He's keeping watch for late-night cleaners, so you're free to focus, explore, worship. Create a pool of saliva by touching the back of your tongue to the roof of your mouth for a minute, then descend on him like a hovercraft. Use your hands and tongue. Wrap one hand around the base of the shaft, slowly move upward, run your palm and fingers over the head, then on the downstroke, twist your hand so you're running it down the opposite side of his penis.

lustylocation

**oh!
oh!
oh!**

orgasmoh!**meter**

riskfactor

A deserted office and you're working late. Your lover thoughtfully stops by with takeout—you take him to Lust Land.

8:25 pm

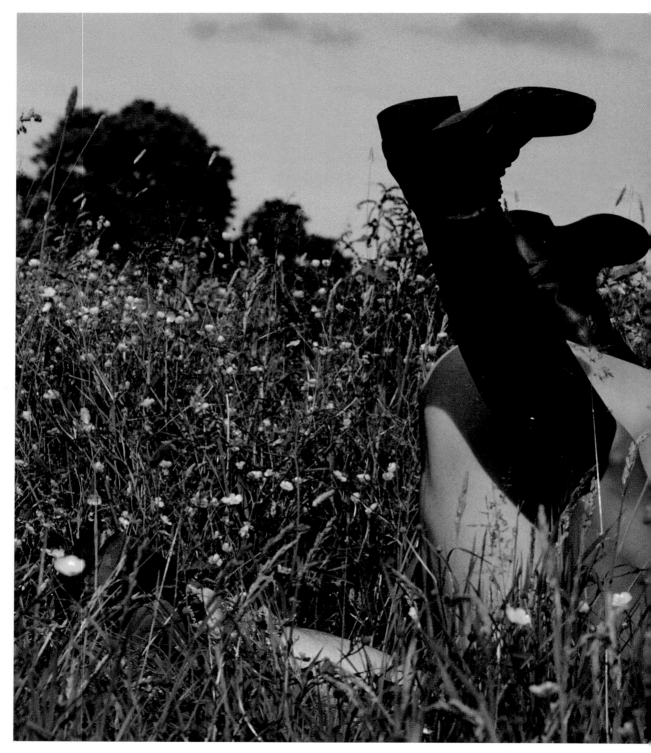

suddenly you decide to ditch the horses and ride each other

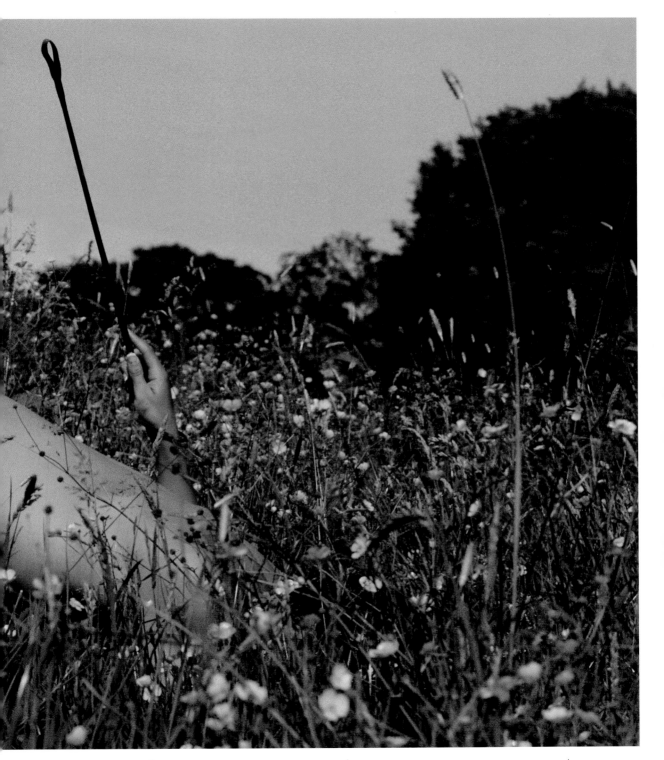

instead. Use the crop to dispense sharp, unexpected spanks.

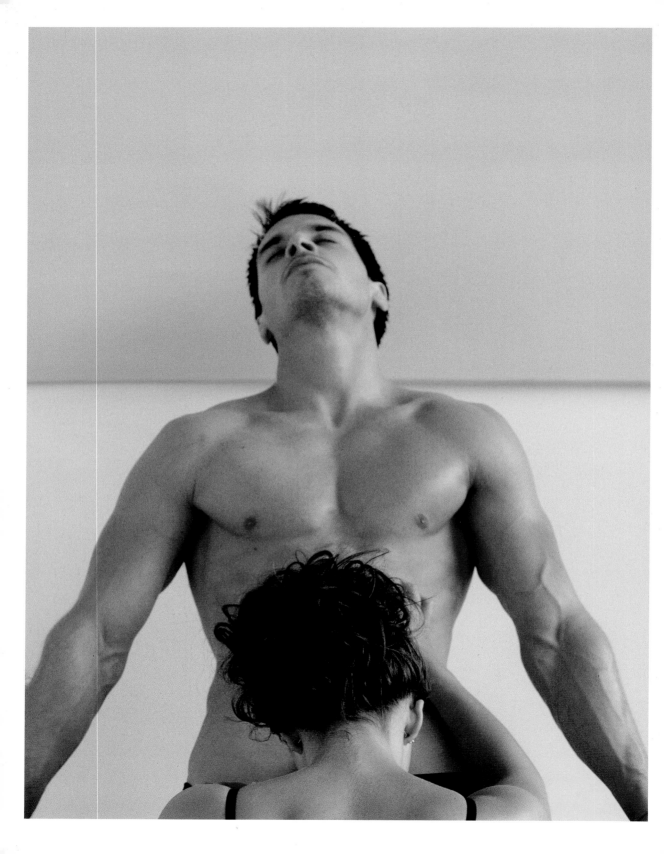

2:10 pm

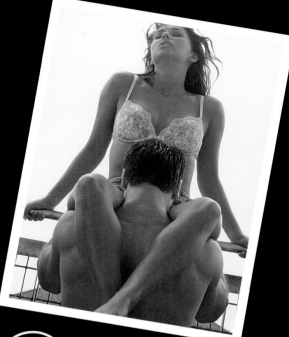

Water and sex go together like masturbation and fantasy. Your private villa has a pool (your parents are away, the resort's deserted)? Time for oral treats! Run your tongue up the raphe (the invisible seam up the center of his scrotum), make slow, torturous circles around the head of his penis, then, holding the flat of your tongue on his frenulum (the stringy bit where the shaft meets the head—the closest equivalent to our clitoris), bob your head up and down. Up her pleasure by maintaining eye contact throughout and describing how she feels, tastes. Stick a finger into her mouth to suck, then, when it's nice and wet, gently insert it into her anus for a bone-rattling, teeth-chattering orgasm.

THE POOL

lustylocation

oh!
oh!
oh!

orgasmoh!**meter**

riskfactor

Just 15 minutes of sunlight produces feel-good serotonin—as does a wet tongue. Take sexy Polaroids to relive it all later.

Quick sex is the BEST sex to..

1

...perfect your hand-job

The humble hand-job comes into its own—literally—during sex in public places. Apart from kissing, using your hands is the lowest-risk sexual activity—and since it's how lots of us masturbate, the genitals respond nicely to the right type of touch. "Right" usually means she should do it harder and he should go softer (it's what each sex is most used to). Not much time? Go for a superfast orgasm for her by positioning her (sitting or standing) in front of you. Rest one palm on the top of her pubic bone and press down firmly, pushing forward, pulling back or moving in circles. Next, insert (well-lubricated) fingers: one inside her vagina, the other in her anus. It's a three-way she won't mind you suggesting—or repeating. Blow him away (in all senses) by trying this technique: Twist your hands in opposite directions as you move up and down (one clockwise, one counterclockwise) or make two fists around his penis, hold them centrally, then move one downward and the other upward. Use one-word questions to ask for feedback (harder? faster?) so he only has to answer yes or no. Keep rhythm constant, building up to a fast speed, then slow it down dramatically before moving back up again. Repeat several times, letting him hover on the brink, before tipping him over with a decided flourish.

2

...rediscover kissing

Romance isn't hijacked by time. A 30-second meeting of mouths is all it takes to turn a quickie into sweet, tender love-making. Kissing is the first thing to go in a long-term relationship: resurrect it and you'll save more than just your sex life. But it's not just dulled passion or overfamiliarity that stops some couples from puckering up. If you actually don't like the way your partner kisses, you'll be more than happy to plunk it in the "things we used to do, but what long-term couple still does?" basket. There's a simple but effective game you can try to fix this. It's called "kisses around the world," and it's best suggested when you're both a little giggly and buzzed and snuggling up after a great night out. Give your partner a little peck, then say "I wonder if people kiss differently around the world? I wonder how Eskimos really kiss. Probably like this..." Then proceed to kiss like an Eskimo, rubbing noses with them. They'll laugh, so it's easy enough from there to say "What about Italians, I think they'd kiss like this..." Before you launch into that one. "How would a French person kiss?", you ask playfully, letting them in on the game. From there it's simply a case of saying "God, that French/Italian/Swedish kiss was hot. Can you do it again?" The next time they kiss you, whisper, "Do it Italian style" and voila! You've transformed an abysmal kisser into a great one—with no one's feelings hurt in the process! If you can't reach each other's lips during certain quickie positions, bite, kiss, or lick the body part closest to you. The more aroused they are, the more dulled their pain receptors—the reason why a nip on the neck feels erotic during sex but just hurts the rest of the time.

3

…up your position portfolio

The average couple alternates between the same three to four positions each time they have intercourse, despite there being more than 600 documented positions to choose from. Before you nominate yourselves for Sad Couple of the Year by fitting right into this category, seek refuge in the fact that virtually all are variants of five basic positions anyway. Besides, certain positions suit certain situations—and moods. Tackling that upside-down one that makes the blood whoosh straight to your head could be just the thing when you're feeling energized and adventurous. Not so appealing when you've got a thumping headache and have just worked a 12-hour day. Quickies provide a great way to try out new, more difficult positions so you can expand your position portfolio. If you don't have to stay at it for long, you're much more likely to attempt something more challenging! Too tired to do anything but missionary? Spice up an old favorite by adding a twist: During intercourse, try mirroring your mouth action to his thrusting, so your tongues are imitating the action of his penis. Once you've mirrored the thrusting speed, you can slow him down or speed him up as you please by simply altering your tongue speed. He'll subconsciously try to keep pace.

4

…make the most of her on top

Given that thrusting is usually *his* job, some women aren't confident masters of the old in-and-out and struggle using just their thigh muscles. Again, far less threatening if she knows it's just a quickie and she's not in it for the long haul; it's much more likely she'll give it the old college try. Next time, get her to make like a frog and squat so her feet are on the floor—it allows much more leverage. Switch her over so she's on top when she's feeling body-proud, horny as hell, and in the mood to be boss. If she needs further convincing, tell her this: rear-entry or any position where she's sitting or squatting over you works best to stimulate a patch of supersensitive skin about two-thirds of the way up from the vaginal entrance on the front wall of the vagina. Nicknamed the "A" spot, it's way up there and hard to reach with fingers, but deep penetration positions sometimes do the trick. Once she's had her (first) orgasm, switch back into missionary. It's got a goody-goody, prissy reputation, but there's a reason why most of us use it a lot of the time: there's full body and eye contact and you can touch faces and hold hands. An intimate ending to a lusty start. Slide a pillow under her hips to turn predictable into predictably pleasurable.

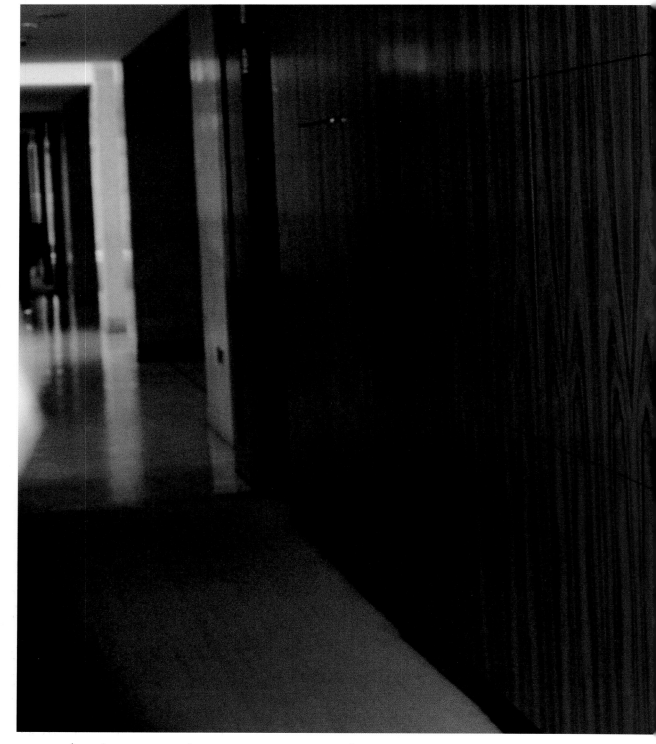

You both spot the girl from the next room sneaking out

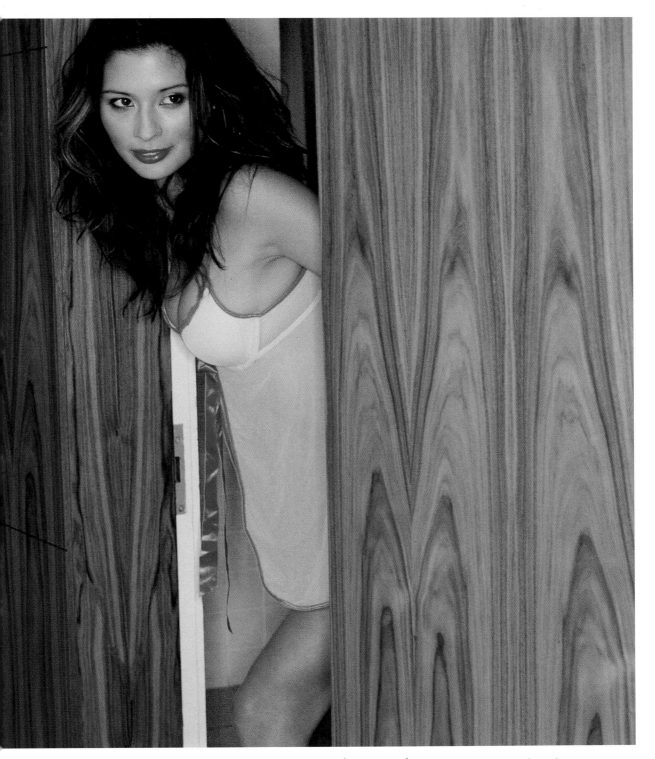

...or ice. Juicy inspiration for that threesome roleplay.

Must
do it now!

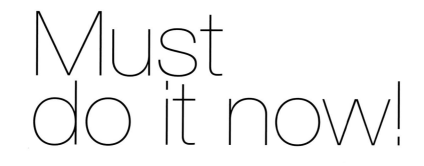

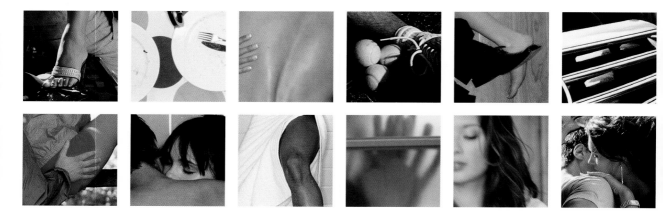

The sudden urge for sex is a powerful force to be resisted only under extreme circumstances (a funeral being the only one I can think of). **Will it really matter if you're five minutes late** or the dishes don't get done? If the kitchen table looks good, go for it. And **won't you be glad you did...**

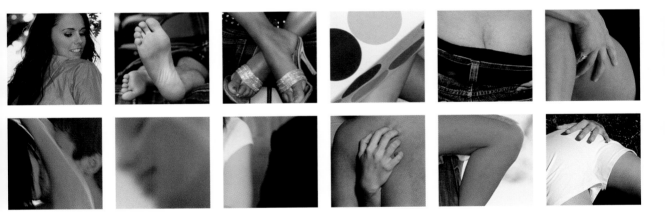

Foreplay that **lasts forever**

People like me have (deliberately) brainwashed men into thinking that foreplay—extended foreplay—is a must for women. I'm not backtracking by encouraging quick sex, simply trying to open up our definition of what foreplay is. Foreplay is anything that gets you both in the mood for sex, sparking your sexual arousal systems. It's commonly thought of as something that you do just before you start having sex—but it needn't be. I strongly recommend couples use "start–stop" sex techniques—turn each other on, then walk away, picking it up again later. You could effectively have ten foreplay "sessions" in a day, without ever following through. What's also interesting is research that shows our need for foreplay appears to

Think foreplay and nearly everyone thinks physical contact. Think more inventively and you realize that a phone call, a look, or even just a word can all make you feel like having sex.

change as we get older. In one study, the majority of men over 35 answered "foreplay" when asked what the best part of sex was. But when women over 35 were asked the same question, they said intercourse. It's a complete turnaround from the standard answers given by those under 35 (most men tend to favor intercourse, most women foreplay). This is great news for both of you. It means your bodies and sexual preferences are changing. Men take longer to get and maintain an erection when older; older women can get turned on more quickly by knowing exactly what does it for them. How to tell how much foreplay is enough? Some sex therapists say listening to a woman's breathing is the best clue to how aroused she is. Moving from normal breathing to a slow, deep, "heavy" pattern usually signals she's ready for intercourse. We tend to shift to "hot and heavy" breathing on approach to orgasm, and plenty of us hold our breath as it happens.

Indulging in public teenage kisses and fumbles might seem juvenile, but it's building your appetite for later. It's a taste-tempting appetizer, designed to hold you over till you dig in to the main course—and dessert.

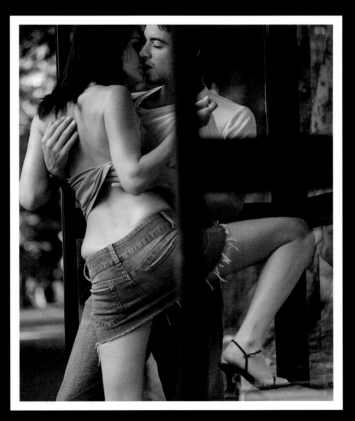

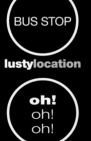

BUS STOP

lustylocation

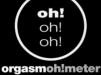

oh!
oh!
oh!

orgasmoh!**meter**

riskfactor

4:45 pm

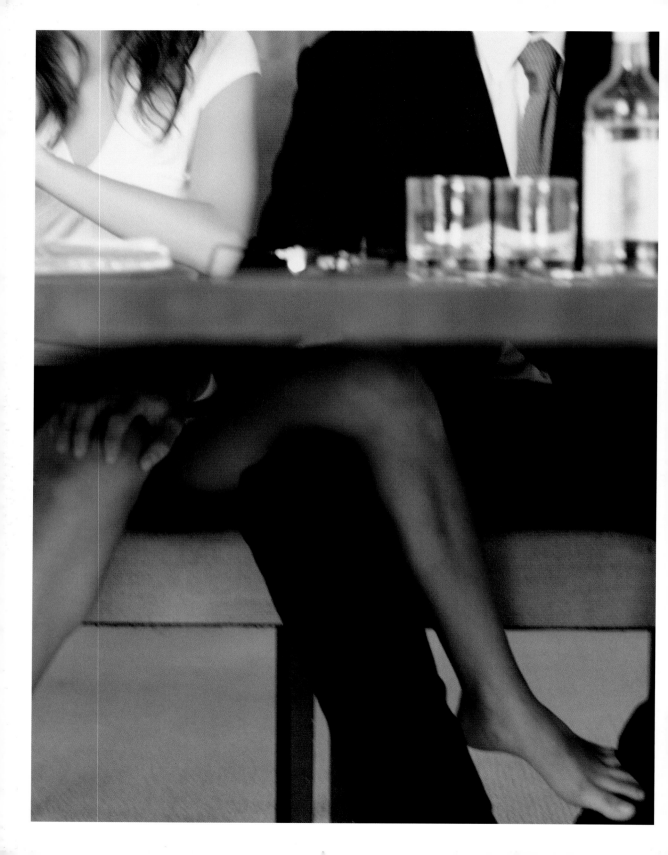

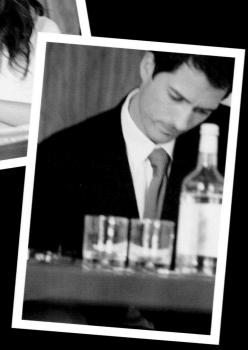

Unless you were planning on resigning and want to go out with a (literal) bang, having sex on the boardroom table during a meeting probably isn't a terribly good idea. But there are ways to send a liberating "up yours" to authority, satisfying the rebellious youth still lurking under the pinstripe suit. Meetings packed with co-workers rather than higher-ups could be worth risking a well-timed, well-executed footsie session, or perhaps even a hand naughtily squeezing his bits or gliding up her stockinged thigh while the others are distracted. Assuming, of course, you're already dating or at least hooking up with the chosen colleague in the stationery closet. Choosing to make a first advance this way will land you with a sexual harassment suit rather than the feel-up you're fantasizing about!

MEETING

lustylocation

oh!
oh!
oh!

orgasmoh!**meter**

riskfactor

If it's above-board above the table, legs askew beneath it go unnoticed. Keep your upper halves businesslike and the bottom can be as impulsive and impetuous as you like.

2:15 pm

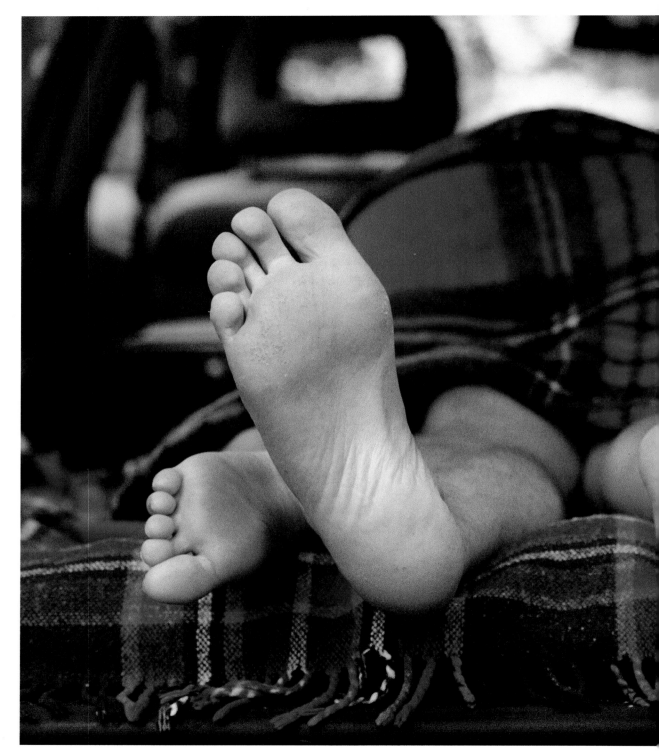

Dull scenery? Well, pull over for a passion pitstop and heat things

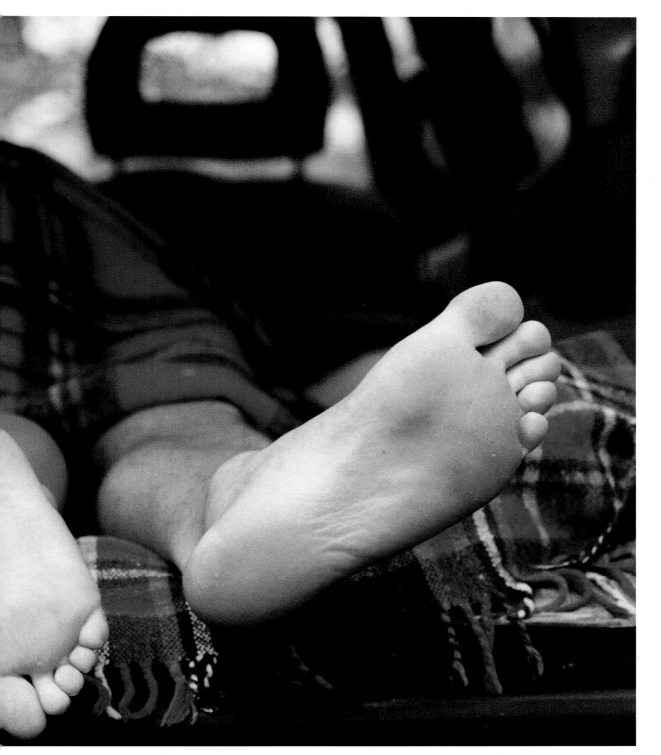

up on the highway with hot, hurried, hellishly good backseat sex.

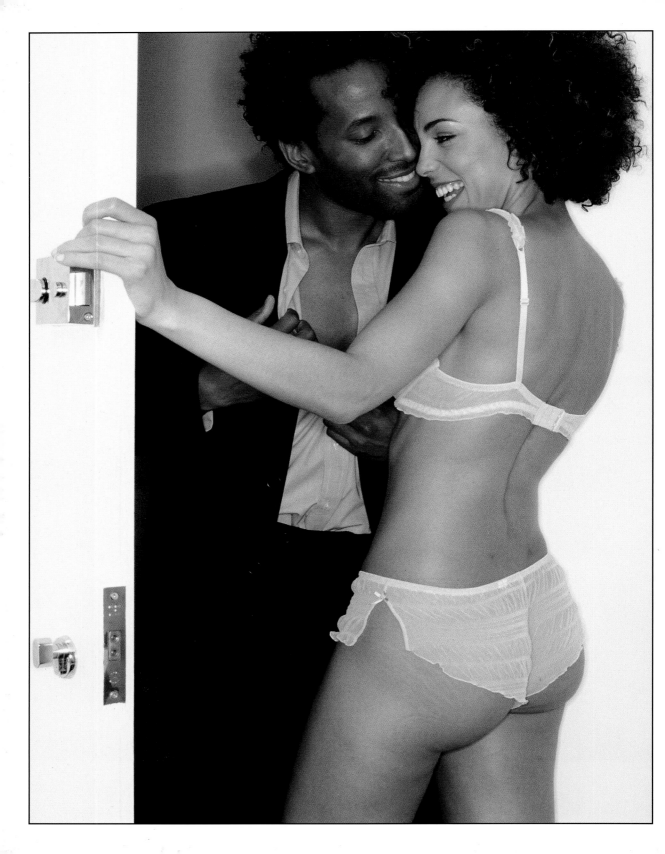

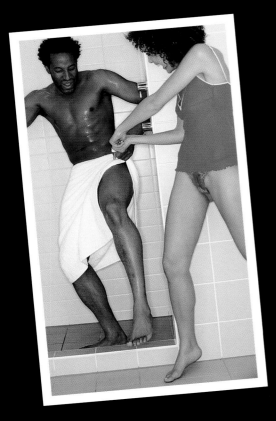

If you're planning on stalling a partner who'd happily quit work and park in front of the TV for life, you probably won't have problems persuading them to postpone their trip to the office for a few pleasure-packed minutes. Workaholics or the dutifully punctual may, however, take a bit of convincing. Ensure that they greet your saucy advances with delight rather than irritation by observing some simple rules. Think before you pounce: is today significant (annual review/ a dreaded meeting where they have to do battle)? If so, forget it; their attention is, and will probably remain, elsewhere. Don't pounce when they're already late: you want them sexually satisfied, not fired. Do nice things to them, rather than expect them to do things to you: it takes a lot less convincing to hang around when you're the one receiving the pleasure. Keep it quick: it's meant to be a tease, not a tantric workout.

HOME

lusty**location**

oh!
oh!
oh!

orgasm**oh!meter**

♡♡♡
♡♡♡

riskfactor

Pounce when they least expect it: fresh from the shower or one hand on the doorknob, about to go to work. You want mere minutes of their time—they'll want you forever.

7:43 am

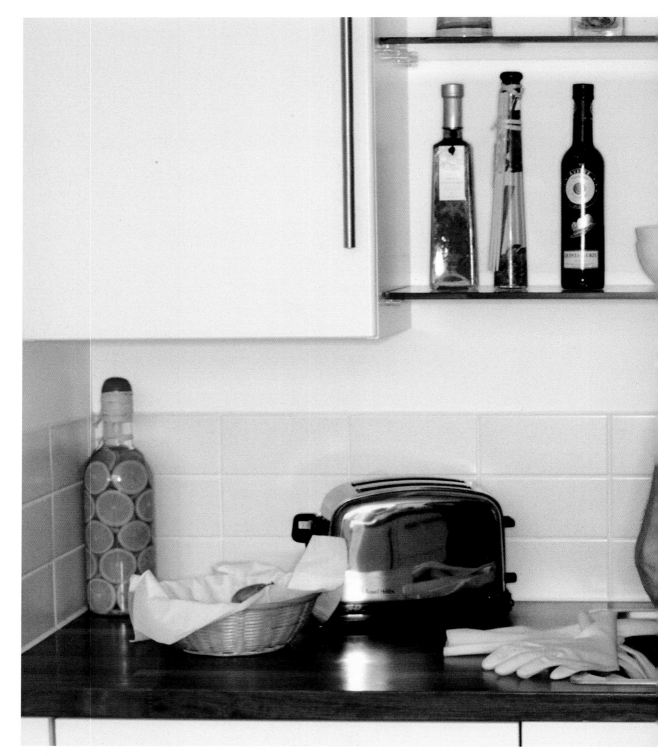

Be a domestic goddess or a naked chef. High benches, wipe-clean

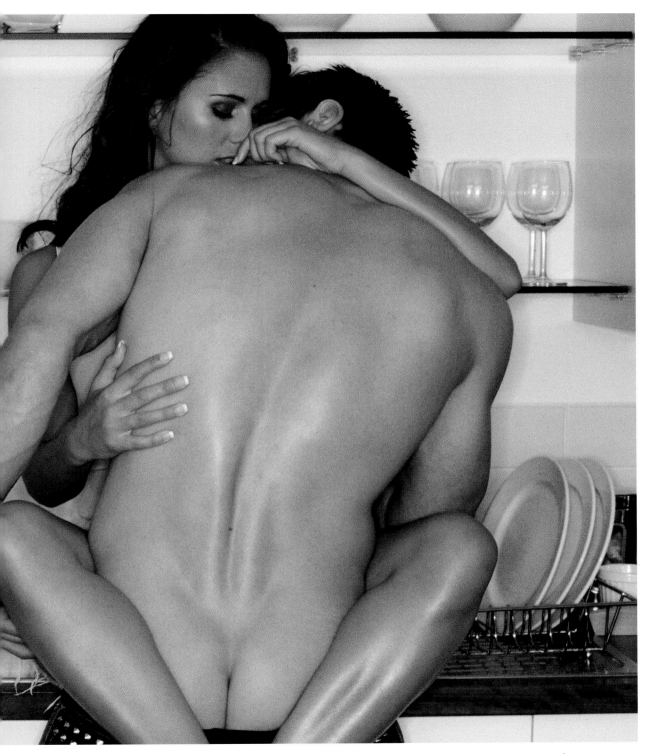

surfaces, and your man elbows-deep in suds. What could be sexier?

Protecting your **private time**

Lack of privacy is a passion-killer. You don't just need time to have sex, you need to be safe from unwanted interruptions when you do, even if it's for five minutes. Whether it's a roommate who seems to be joined to you by an invisible rubber band, constant phone calls from a bored buddy, or kids barging in whenever they damn well feel like it, lack of private time together won't just thwart your sex life, it'll kill your relationship, too. Be sexually selfish: guard time together ferociously and remind yourselves that the sexually satisfied make happier friends, parents, and colleagues. Put a lock on the bedroom door and use it. Enforce bedtime for kids and a rule that everyone in the family knocks and waits for an answer before entering

If you must, lie to buy yourselves private time! You can't come to dinner because you've got a visitor arriving from overseas (that box of sex toys you ordered) or you have to finish a work assignment (playing out a boss-secretary sex fantasy).

a bedroom. Put a radio next to the bed to mute the sounds of sex; turn phones off when it's "your" time. Maximize precious time alone by turning yourselves on quickly: have a series of code words that remind you of previous lusty encounters. "Sue's bathroom" whispered into her ear as she's making the kids' beds conjures up memories of you taking her from behind at a party; "rubber" reminds him of what you did after you pulled on those latex gloves. When your partner touches you with wicked intent, stop thinking and start feeling. Concentrating on their touch, on what's happening right now, cuts off any brain protestations of why you shouldn't be having sex. Left to its own devices, your body is usually more than happy to say "yes" to potential pleasure.

Set up a lifestyle that allows you to steal intimate moments. Be on red alert for situations with a low risk of public exposure and zero chance of interruption. It takes mere seconds to have a passionate encounter.

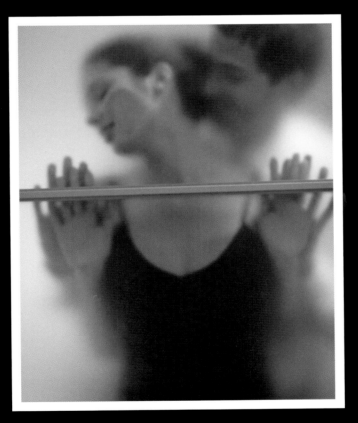

THE GYM
lustylocation

oh!
oh!
oh!
orgasm**oh!meter**

riskfactor

4:45 pm

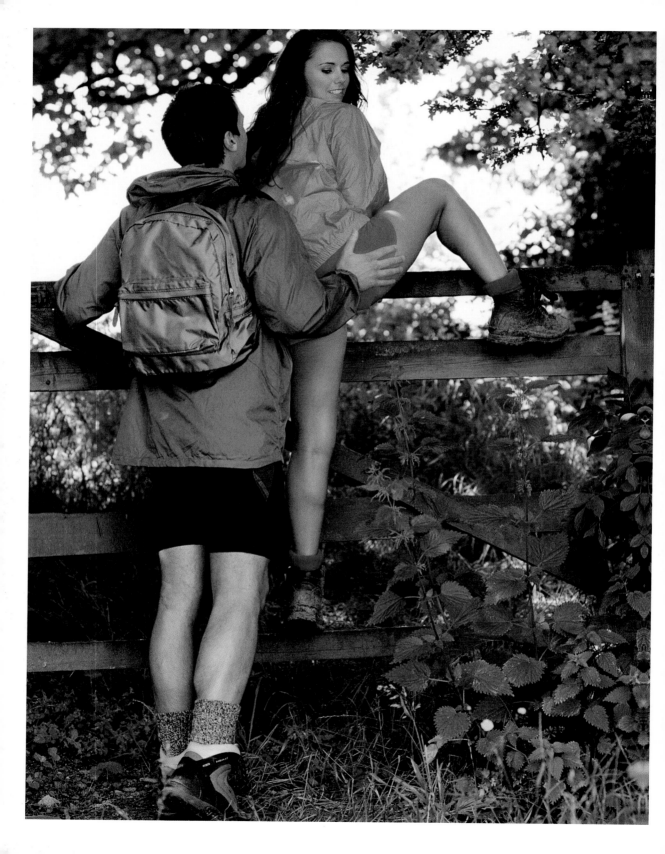

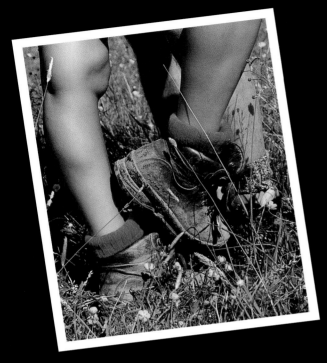

Heading out for a romantic, hand-in-hand stroll through the countryside is a favorite new-couple pastime. Happily (unlike kissing, sex three times a day, and staying up till six making out), it's one of the few activities most couples are still doing ten years into the relationship. But instead of making it the precursor to that boozy Sunday lunch, teeter out afterward, when you're feeling warm and fuzzy, inhibitions pleasantly dulled by that wonderful bottle of red you consumed. Stake out a likely place beforehand (a tree-dense route that isn't terribly popular, with plenty of secret clearings where you won't be disturbed), then indulge in a little alfresco. Even if you do exactly the same things you do in that comfy marital bed at home, just taking it outdoors adds the frisson that tends to fade over time.

HIKING

lustylocation

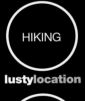

oh!
oh!
oh!

orgasmoh!**meter**

riskfactor

Quickies aren't a pale imitation of "real" sex. They're an inspired way to add longed-for spice and spontaneity.

10:30 am

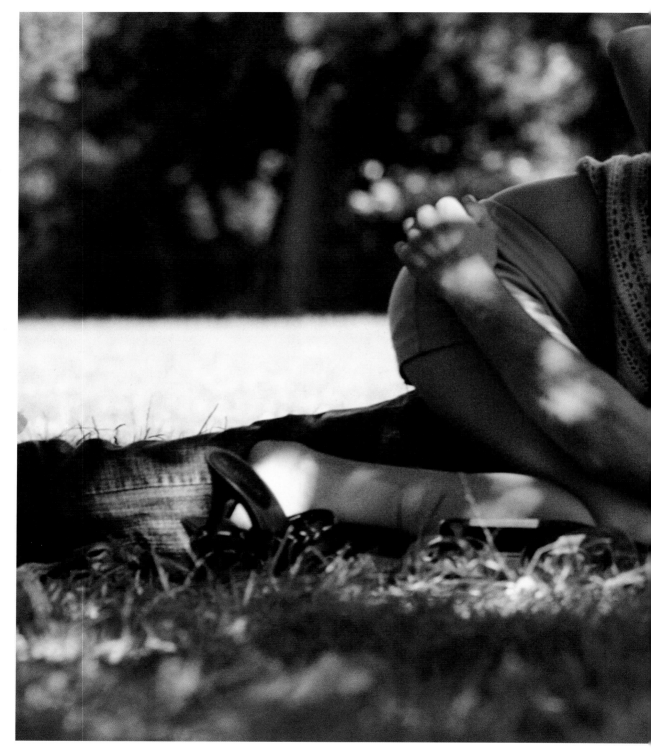

Pounce in the park with a healthy disregard for grass stains and

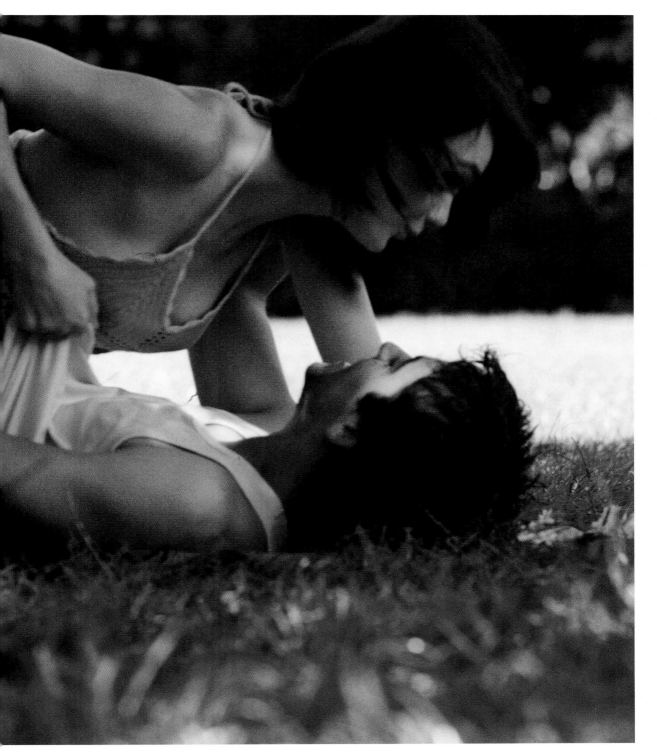

telltale twigs protruding from your hair. Playful is provocative.

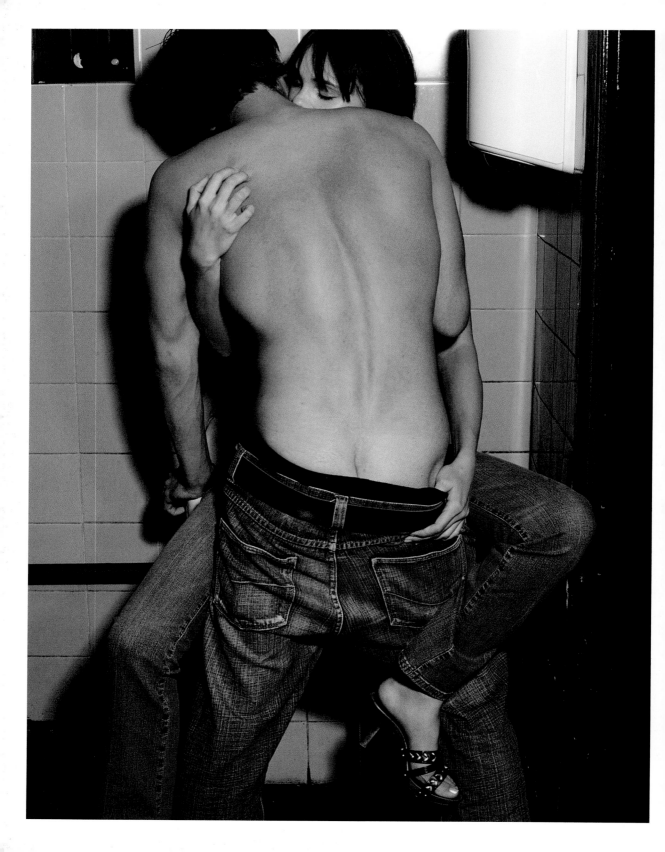

You're out with friends, laughing and living it up, when you look across at your partner and realize, even in a packed room of attractive strangers, they're the person you'd choose to go home with every time. You catch their eye and give a tiny, imperceptible nod toward the "restroom" sign. They smile, nod back, and follow within a few minutes...

With a three-minute deadline, you're more inclined to let loose and dive in enthusiastically, greedily devouring whatever flesh you can get your hands and mouth on. It's also easier to act out a sexy scene or fantasy in an unfamiliar location. Restrooms are associated with drug-use and illicit sex, so sex takes on an edgy, dangerous feel (even if you have nothing to fear but the embarrassment of being caught). Scorching, peppery—a total sexual recharge.

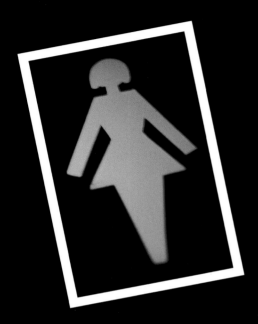

REST-
ROOM

lustylocation

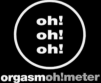

oh!
oh!
oh!

orgasmoh!**meter**

♥♥♥
♥♥

riskfactor

Disappear to the loo and do more than touch-up your makeup. The slightly sordid, sleazy surroundings supersize your sex drive.

12:40 pm

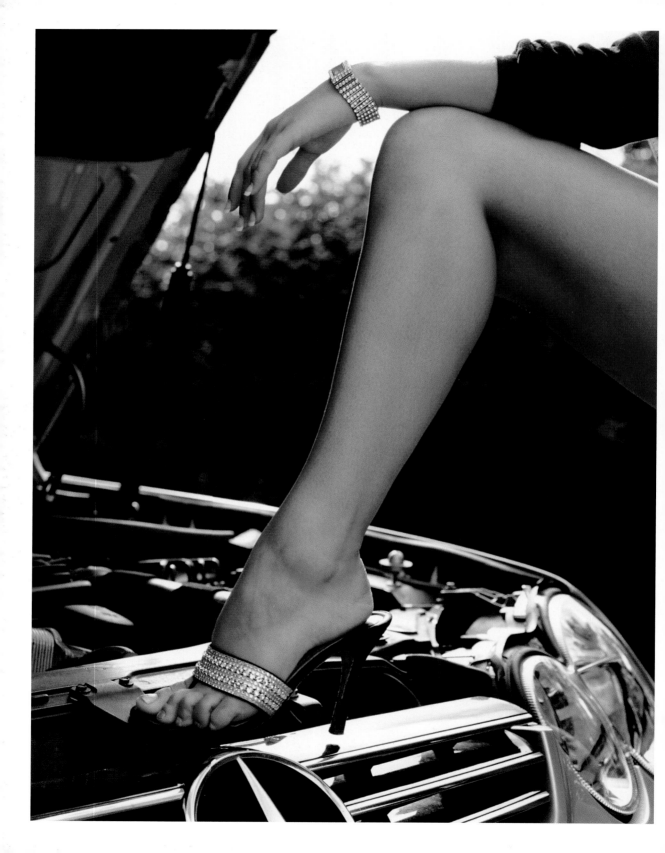

11:45 am

It's all about the situation: he's immune to seeing you naked pre-bedtime, but a flash of thigh by the roadside is unexpectedly voyeuristic. The secret to loving lustily long-term is to surprise each other sexually. Within a year of saying "I do," most couples are saying "I don't want to." Why? No variety = no interest. Sex on the hood of the car might seem raw and unromantic when you have a big, soft bed to roll around in, but contrast is the key.

ROADSIDE

lustylocation

oh!
oh!
oh!

orgasmoh!meter

riskfactor

Stranded, bored, and waiting for the tow truck, an innocent kiss turns into a smoldering smooch. Surely the mechanic has seen it all before?

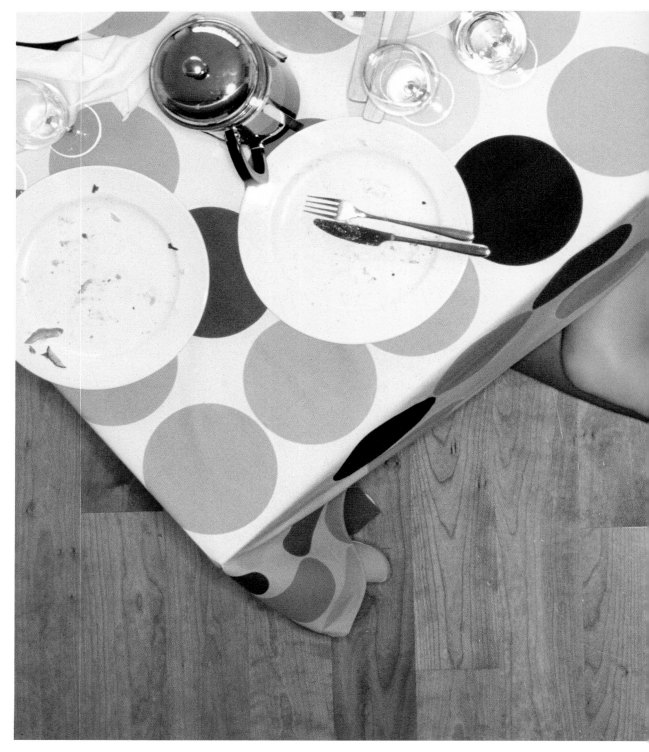

Tipsy at a friend's dinner party, you disappear under

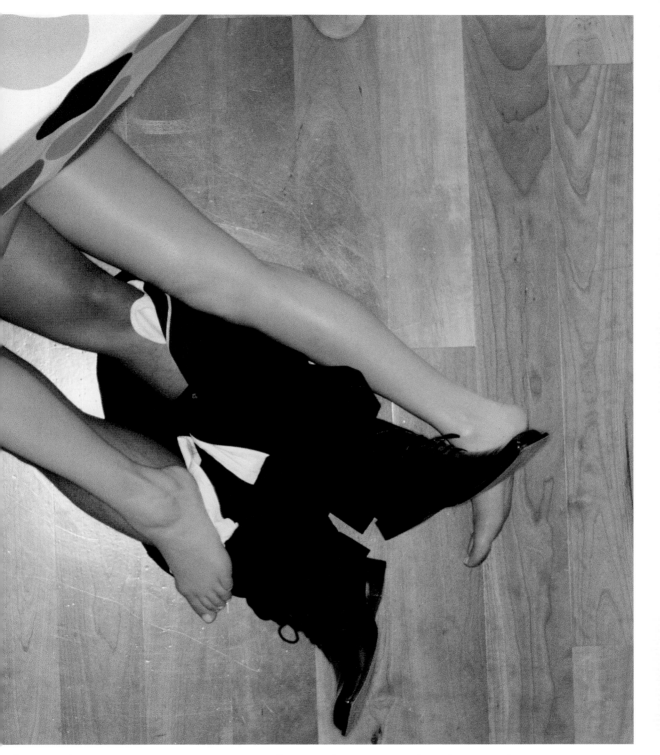

he table. You did offer to help them with the dishes!

Three minutes to spare

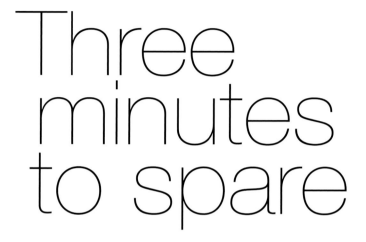

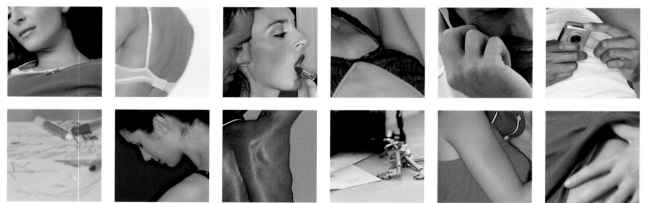

No time for sex? Are you sure? Think of all those **wasted minutes** waiting for a cab to arrive, yawning through the commercials, the coffee break you take as you wade through paperwork. **Grab it while you can and you might find yourselves making time to grab each other.**

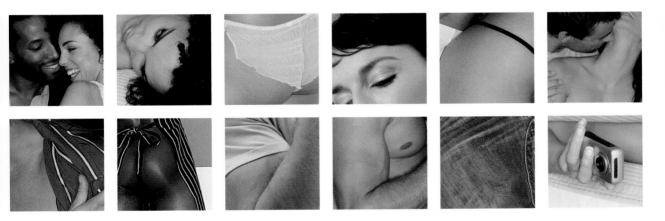

Making time for making whoopee

To get more sex, stop wasting time on unimportant things. We budget our money and are aware of (or at least pretend to be) where each penny disappears to. But we're far less careful with our time. It's seriously worth keeping a time diary for two days during the week and one weekend to identify time-wasters. Write down what you're doing and how long you're spending on it. Include everything: phone calls, chores, texting, emails, TV time, sleep time, eating time, couple time, sex time, socializing, exercise, chores, and work. Then take a look at how you can free up time for nicer things... like sex! Get in the habit of screening calls and keeping return calls to a limit. If possible, hire a cleaner. Have a bank

We'll schedule in fun times with friends but baulk at the idea of planned sex time. The perception is if sex isn't spontaneous, it's not enjoyable. But if this is true, how come we enjoy dinner out, when the restaurant was booked a week in advance?

of reliable babysitters and buy a baby monitor so you can keep tabs on what's happening elsewhere while you're up to no good in the other room. Cut down your TV time. Shop online, get takeout, cook extra and freeze it. Invest in labor-saving devices like a dishwasher. Slot in sex time and one "date" per week, just the two of you. You don't have to have sex during "sex time," just create an opportunity for the two of you to be alone together. Even if you end up changing the time or day you'd assigned, you've officially blocked off a period of time and are much more likely to make an effort to ensure that it happens than if you'd left it in the lap of the lazy Time Gods. When it's time for your date, both make an effort to look good. Clichéd advice, perhaps, but if you actually do it, it makes a difference.

The theater beckons, but then so does the carpet. You're both glammed up, suited and booted— irresistible to each other. Give in to mutual appreciation. In the time it takes for a cab to come, you both could, too.

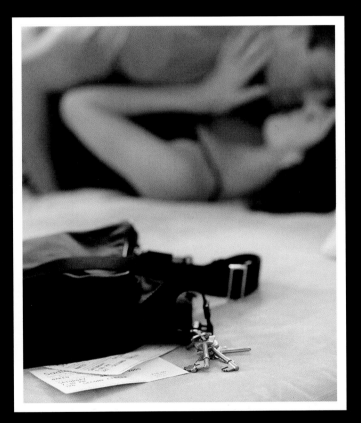

PRE-THEATER

lustylocation

oh!
oh!
oh!

orgasm**oh!**meter

♡♡♡
♡♡

riskfactor

7:45 pm

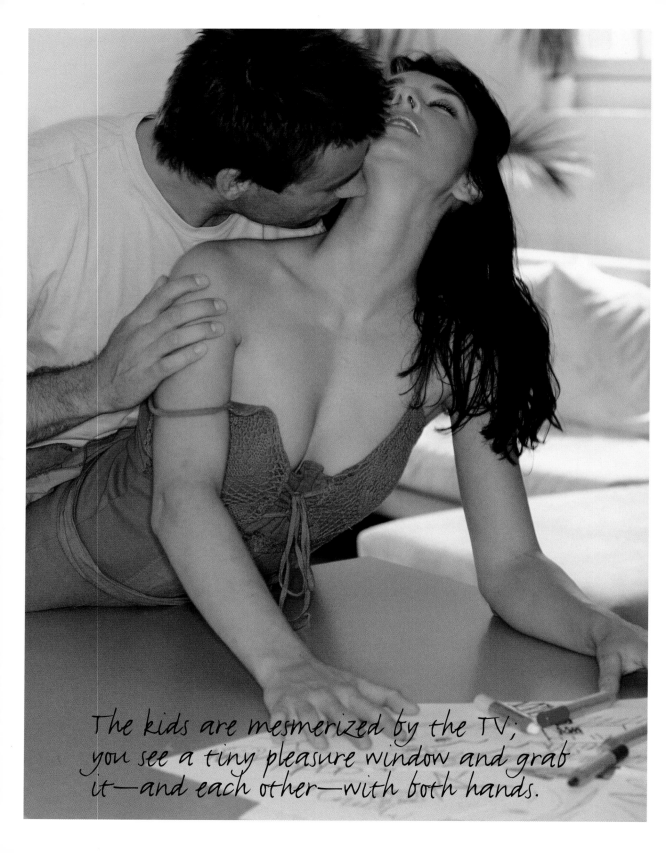

The kids are mesmerized by the TV; you see a tiny pleasure window and grab it—and each other—with both hands.

4:30 pm

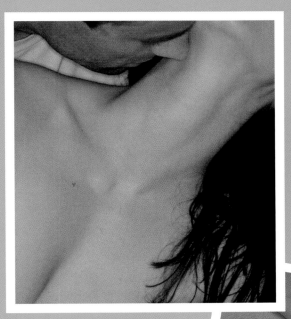

Happy parents means happy kids means you shouldn't feel the slightest bit guilty for stealing frequent "Mommy–Daddy alone" moments. Disappear into the bathroom for a quick oral session, linger near the sink for a long, juicy kiss. If you feel too frazzled, burdened, or burned out for sex, do sensual things instead. A mini-massage, brushing each other's hair, sharing a bath—they feel great, and the more relaxed your body and mind, the more likely you are to feel that delicious desire tingle.

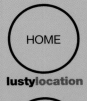

lustylocation

HOME

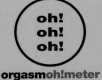

orgasmoh!**meter**

oh!
oh!
oh!

riskfactor

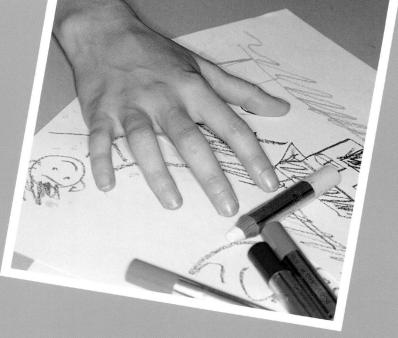

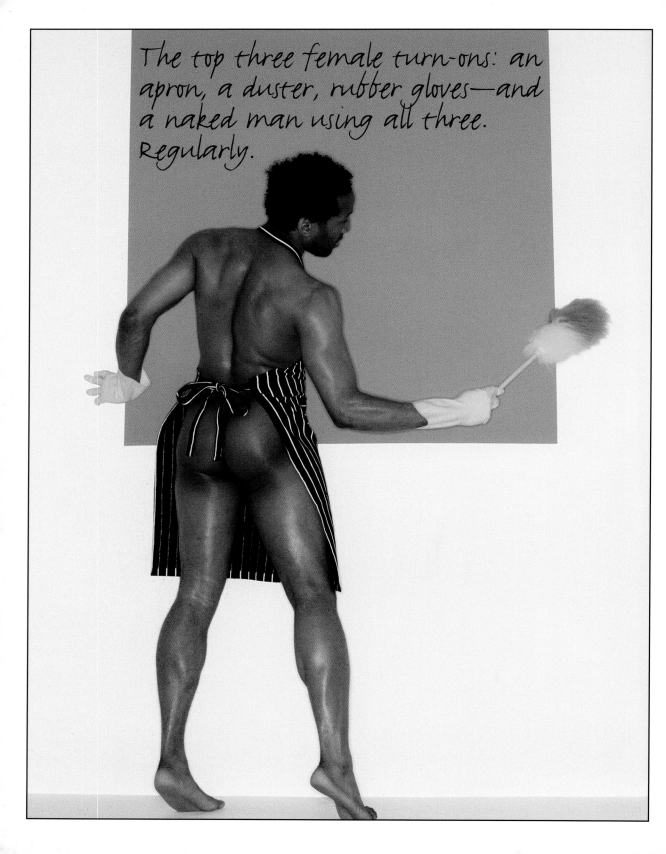

The top three female turn-ons: an apron, a duster, rubber gloves—and a naked man using all three. Regularly.

If the quickest way to a man's heart is through his stomach, the quickest way to a woman's crotch is doing the dishes after she cooks for you. Housework isn't her job—and men who believe it is are deeply unsexy. You both make the mess, both clean it up. Treating her like a cleaner means resentment, and we all know what comes of that: neither of you two! The more housework the man does, the more sex the couple has. We all need chill-out time in order to feel sexy. Sending her off for a bath while you clean up can do more for your sex life than sixty Kama-Sutra-style positions.

HOME

lustylocation

oh!
oh!
oh!

orgasmoh!**meter**

♡ ♡ ♡
♡ ♡

riskfactor

9:30 am

quick ways to climax

tip-**him**-over tricks

❤ **Hold a vibrator** on your cheek or on his testicles as you're fellating him ❤ **Tie him up**—he's often the sexual instigator, so removing power is a huge turn-on ❤ **Add clothes to a naked body**—high heels, a push-up bra ❤ **Maintain eye contact** as you touch, suck, lick him ❤ **Watch an erotic movie together** with the rule that neither of you is allowed to take your eyes off the screen, no matter what's going on off-screen ❤ **Touch yourself** while he's making love to you—caress your breasts, dip your fingers inside, stroke your clitoris ❤ Throw in some **dirty talk** ❤ **Use the head of his penis** to stimulate your nipples and clitoris ❤ **Do it rear-entry** so he can penetrate as deeply as possible ❤ **Insert a well-lubricated finger** up his bottom ❤ Detail his **favorite fantasy** ❤ **Get him on all fours**, then slide underneath to give him oral sex ❤ **Swirl your tongue** over his testicles to make him feel like *all* of him is involved ❤ **You lie back**, head on the pillow, he hovers above you, his weight on his arms, **thrusting into your mouth.**

treat tricks

❤ **Masturbate for him**—as he instructs you. He can't touch, but he can tell you where and how and how long you're to touch yourself. An astute lover will know when you're close to orgasm and get you to stop or switch stimulation to prolong the floor show.

❤ **Make him put on your lacy, satiny French panties** Females get to wear all sorts of different clothes and fabrics, but silk boxers are about as sexy as it gets for the feel of slippery fabric against male skin. Jokingly get him to try on your panties (buy a big pair if you're tiny and he's not), then start masturbating him through the fabric, moving on to lick and mock-bite up and down the sides of his erection. If he starts to freak, don't panic. The whole experience feels so good, he's worried it means he's gay. Reassure him it doesn't. It's simply a naughty, "forbidden" experience that you're getting off on as well.

tip-**her**-over tricks

❤ **Add a blindfold**—females are more sensation-seeking and less visual than men. Deprived of sight, she'll **focus on feeling**, which is always a very good thing ❤ Get her to **lick your palm** to show you what **tongue strokes excite her most** ❤ **Spread her arms wide** or hold both wrists together over her head, before **caressing her breasts**. They're more sensitive when the skin around them is taut ❤ **Use three fingers to stimulate her**: rub the two outside fingers down the edges of the vaginal lips, working externally, then part her gently and use the middle finger on her clitoris ❤ **Get her to stand while you kneel before her**, exciting those slave/master fantasies as you give her oral ❤ **Turn on an erotic movie** featuring women making love to women. It's most females' **secret sex fantasy**, and being ordered to indulge removes embarrassment ❤ **Penetrate from behind**, pull back and **slap her on the fleshy part of her bottom** with the back of a hairbrush (test the strength on your hand first) ❤ **Pinch or tweak** her nipples *hard*, just as she's about to climax.

treat tricks

❤ **Get her to watch herself during phone sex.** Ask her to sit in front of a full-length mirror during the call. As you tell her what to do—sit with legs apart, take her top off, touch herself—she watches the show. She gets to see what your eyes are normally treated to, boosting body image and sexing up future erotic encounters.

❤ **Up the intensity of oral sensation** by getting her to pull her knees up to her chest. Alternatively, get her to hold the fleshy part of the pubic mound, pushing it up and away (toward her tummy), to expose the clitoris and make it easier for you to work on. Flatten your tongue rather than use the tip, keep the whole area wet, and make big, slow licks, maintaining a steady rhythm. Lots of women have a favorite "side" to the clitoris—concentrate stimulation on either side and ask her to rate which is hers.

Sparky sex in **60 seconds**

Give me 60 seconds and I'll transform your sex life. OK, I might need some of those 60 seconds throughout the week, but I pretty much guarantee if you mix a few of these simple, minute-long sex tricks into your usual routine, life will seem a whole lot sparklier. They're low-effort, low-stress sex enhancers that work on the premise of tease: a little of something you want makes you want a whole lot more of it. The idea is to keep you both simmering: thinking frequently and fondly about sex with each other, even while apart. I'll start by giving you some suggestions, but you'll see you can incorporate virtually anything in this book (or your existing repertoire) to fit the formula. Here goes... Leave sex letters as well

There's just one rule: you must mean what you say and follow through with your promise at some point. Six, seconds-long sex tricks strung out over three days—with no relief—turns a fervid tease into a rather unpleasant torture.

as love letters ("Do you know how hot you are?" as well as "Love you, honey"); Both perfect the 30-second head-job—unzip jeans or slide panties aside, wrap lips softly around his penis, or dispense one, long lick on her inner labia, gently do whatever their favorite thing is for 30 seconds, then... stop; Take his hand and put it up your skirt while you're out, for him to find you're naked underneath; Give her a champagne kiss by dribbling a little, bit by bit, from your mouth into hers; Grab some bedside lubricant, then lower yourself on his morning glory for one minute and *only* 15 slow, grinding thrusts; Splurge on a sexy French erotic flick, find the sexiest part, then tease her by playing just one or two minutes; Put on a minute-long floor show and show him just how fabulous your new vibrator really is.

You're absorbed in getting ready for a dinner out, he's transfixed by the process. Sensational lingerie, freshly washed hair, a slick of gloss on lips he instantly, desperately wants to smudge... too bad he's not allowed. Till later.

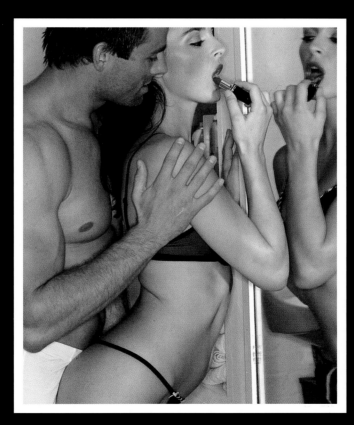

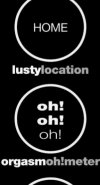

HOME

lustylocation

oh!
oh!
oh!

orgasm**oh!**meter

riskfactor

7:10 pm

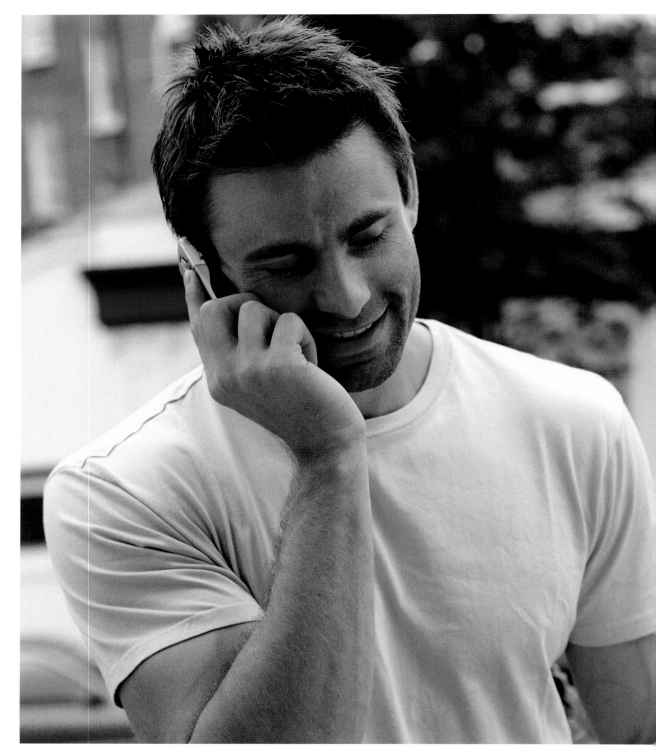

Call him when masturbating with a stroke-by-stroke

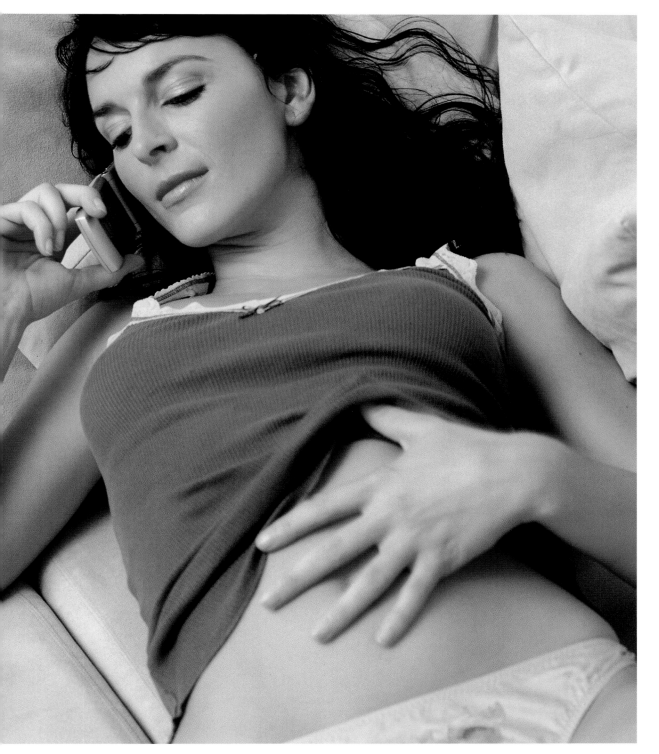

commentary. High arousal without so much as a touch.

Just
for kicks

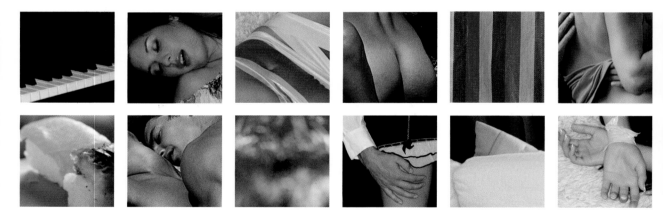

The need to be naughty is something to be encouraged, not resisted. Fancy **smearing food** instead of eating it? **Devouring her** instead of that book? **Tying your partner up** rather than tying them down to their promise of doing your tax return? Impish urges, sinful thoughts, devilish desire—**wicked works**.

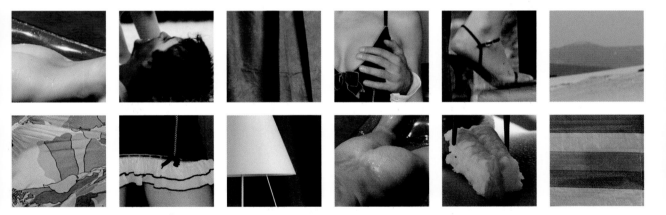

Enticing her to try the **kinky stuff**

So you have the urge to be wicked and get a bit kinky, but while *you* want to be experimental, your partner might need a little persuasion. How and when do you approach the subject? Whether it be a hot colleague or a long-term lover you'd love to get kinky with, there are things you can do to virtually guarantee success. Number 1 rule: don't "kink" too quickly. It's usually a good idea to wait until the second month you and your girlfriend have been having sex before dropping a super-naughty suggestion. She'll be more comfortable with you and less likely to run for the door. Make her feel it's partly her fault by pitching it as something you've never done with anyone else or wanted to… but she's soooo sexy, you

Start off small instead of diving straight in with a weird one. Suggesting you tie her to the bedposts with her stockings is acceptable; pulling on a mask and emerging from the closet, whip in hand, probably isn't.

can't help but imagine what it would be like. Keep it light-hearted—the more playful you are, the less freaked she'll be (and if she looks at you like you've just asked for a threesome with her grandma, you can pretend you were kidding). Don't push the issue if it's clear she doesn't want to go there; if she does agree, make it clear she can stop the play at any point if she doesn't enjoy it. Load on the compliments afterward—both sexual and emotional— and she's putty in your hands for those other dozen suggestions you have on your list! A well-educated girlfriend won't need much persuading—women with college degrees are more likely to engage in both oral and anal sex—and a girl with a Ph.D. is twice as likely to be interested in a one-night stand!

The secret to successful, seductive persuasion is making the encounter both sexy and safe. Do some sleuthing: search for secluded, tucked-away hideaways, far from the public gaze.

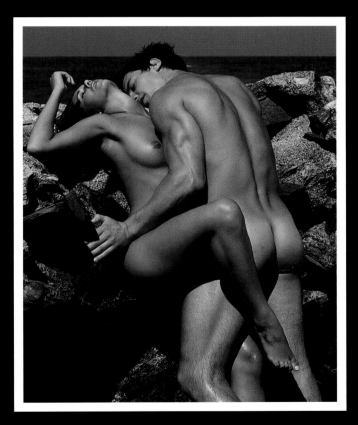

ROCKS

lustylocation

oh!
oh!
oh!

orgasmoh!meter

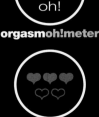

riskfactor

1:45 pm

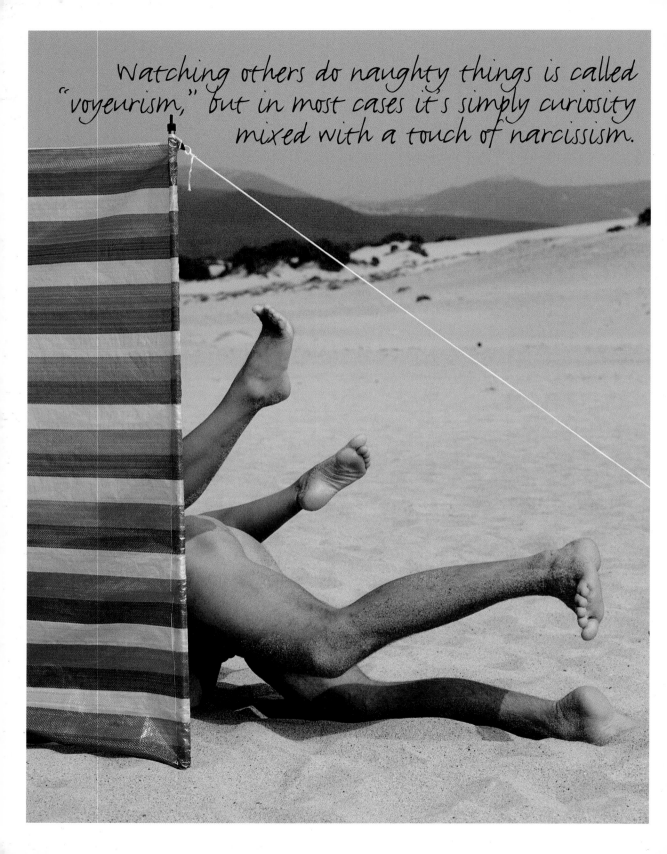

Watching others do naughty things is called "voyeurism," but in most cases it's simply curiosity mixed with a touch of narcissism.

11:45 am

Most people, stumbling across a couple having sex in semi-public, would be hard-pressed not to sneak a rather l-o-n-g peek before discreetly leaving or announcing their presence. The reason why is because we rarely, if ever, get to see real people having sex because it's kept hidden and private. By watching, we get to see what we probably look like having sex— and fantasize about how much better we'd perform under the same circumstances. If you're aware you're providing the entertainment and continue, you officially become an "exhibitionist." Your motivation is also tinged with narcissism—others are admiring you, envious of your sexual skills and desperately wishing they were the person you were making love to. A good, healthy ego-boost all around, really!

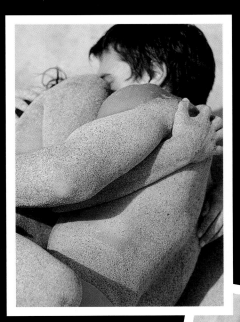

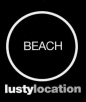

BEACH

lustylocation

oh!
oh!
oh!

orgasmoh!**meter**

riskfactor

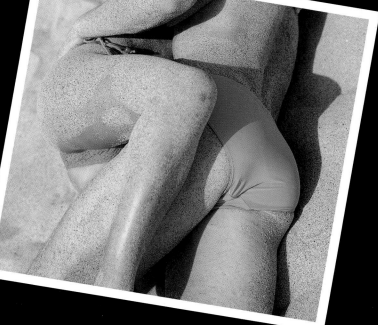

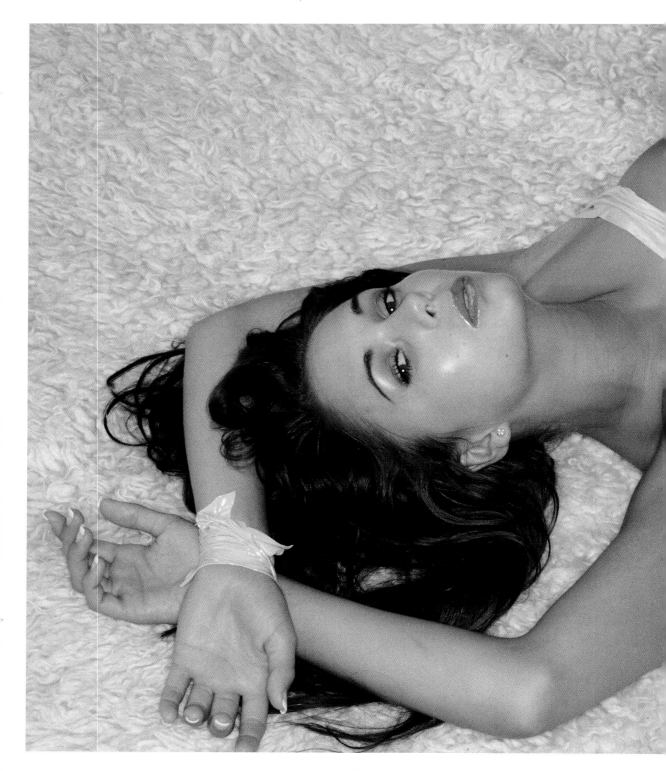

Tousled and trussed, using pink bondage tape rather than rope,

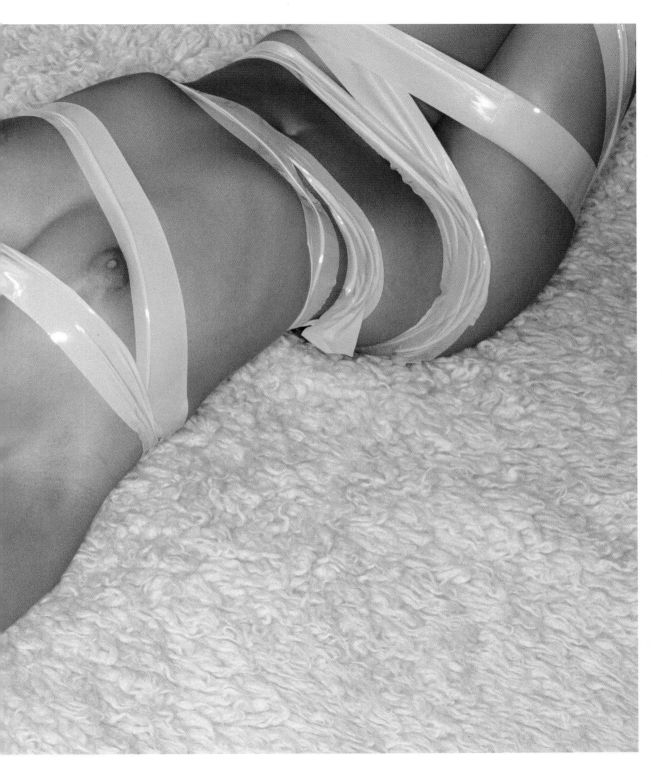

you've prettily surrendered power—to become his ultimate fantasy.

Saucier, spicier sex

dirty talk

Most men beat women hands down when it comes to talking dirty. All those men's mags have made you **immune to "bad" words** and you really don't care if what you say sounds clichéd or cheesy, because you know dirty talk always sounds ridiculous when taken out of context (and often while in it). But do you care if you sound like a pathetically stilted porn extra? Nah! You're too busy enjoying the effect your words are having on both of you! Pay attention, girls, and push embarrassment to one side. **Saying dirty things** to each other, or describing **current, future, or imaginary action**, excites most of us because it's something "nice"

myself disappear inside you"). In fact, doing nothing but describing the sex you're having as you're having it is a good place to start. Move on to telling them **what you're about to do, just before you do it** and you're a teensy step from describing lusciously lewd fantasies out loud. Slow down, add drama, perfect your timing, and build in lots of detail, and you'll be rivaling those husky phone-sex operators before you know it!

Don't know what to say? **Steal stuff from erotic books and magazines**. Your partner won't know (or care). Pay attention during movies that turn you on: which words and phrases do it for you, and which don't?

If you're struggling to use "naughty" words or simply talk out loud during sex, learn to link noise and desire by talking dirty out loud to yourself while masturbating.

people don't do. "Nice" girls don't swear or get horny, and "nice" boys pretend not to notice if we do (yeah, right). Lots of us make love in silence, so any sort of noise is mildly shocking. And describing out loud what the two of you are up to is particularly risqué.

As a general rule, **match your dirty talk to theirs**. While it's often the case that the geeky, "innocent" types want the dirtiest obscenities whispered, it's easy to offend and hard to find just the right balance for erotic effect. Start safe and low-key. Dirty talk doesn't even have to be dirty—it can simply be observational ("**I'm watching**

Start an **erotic diary** and write down all the sexy phrases and scenarios that arouse you. Rather than startle your lover by breaking a stoic silence with an unexpected frantic flow of sex talk, start off by simply moaning during sex. Move on to simple one-sentence descriptions ("God, that feels good"), then comment on what's happening. Try **reliving your last steamy session out loud** ("Remember when you..."), or play a game where you both start with a provocative sentence ("We're at your parents' for lunch and they've gone out to get some milk"), leaving the other to add the next sentence to **build a fantasy**.

be anal about better, deeper orgasms

Want to make each other climax more quickly and intensely? Want to add **instant erotic thrill and adventure**? Well, what's the body part with the highest concentration of nerve endings, besides the genitals? That's right… your bottom! Worried that it's "wrong" or unnatural? Well, famous sexpert Alfred Kinsey said the only unnatural sex act was the one you can't perform—a healthy attitude to adopt (within reason, obviously!). **Plenty who thought they wouldn't like bottom play end up converts once they've tried it**. Game to give it a try? Start by either using your tongue (rimming) to explore each other anally, or use a finger to see how

free hand to give him **a fierce, frenzied orgasm**. Stimulate the anus with your mouth. (If you're squeamish, use a little piece of plastic wrap.) If you're ready to try anal intercourse, it's good for her to orgasm beforehand (it relaxes the muscles) and it's essential she knows saying "stop" will result in your doing just that. Using lots of lube, insert a finger, then gradually your penis, waiting for her permission at each step. If she contracts her muscles, reassure her she's in control. Once you're fully inserted (which may take several sessions), **thrust slow and shallow** to begin with—and don't be surprised if you ejaculate way before you expected to! It's

It's often neglected sexually for lots of (often quite silly) reasons, but if you don't try some form of anal stimulation at least once, you are seriously missing out.

you like it. Feeling a bit panicked about potential pain? Don't be. If you take your time, wait for your muscles to relax, use buckets of lubrication, take baby steps, and provide constant feedback, you will be fine. Promise! **Rub your fingertip around the outside of the anus in a gentle, circular motion**. When the muscles relax, insert it a tiny way, constantly checking that it's OK with your partner. Once your finger is fully inserted, move it in a circular, rather than in-out motion. For him, **stimulate his G-spot** by moving your finger in a "come here" motion toward his belly button and masturbate him with your

not just "forbidden" sex, the anal canal is extremely tight. If anal sex is your **New Favorite Thing**, you need to be aware that the rectum contains bacteria that can cause serious infections in the vagina. Remove condoms and wash fingers, toys, and body parts with antibacterial soap before vaginal love-making. Condoms should protect you against HIV, hepatitis, and other infections but, personally, it's so high-risk, I'd avoid having anal intercourse with anyone I didn't trust implicitly or who hadn't been tested for most STDs. Protect yourself against parasitic infections during rimming by using that little bit of plastic wrap.

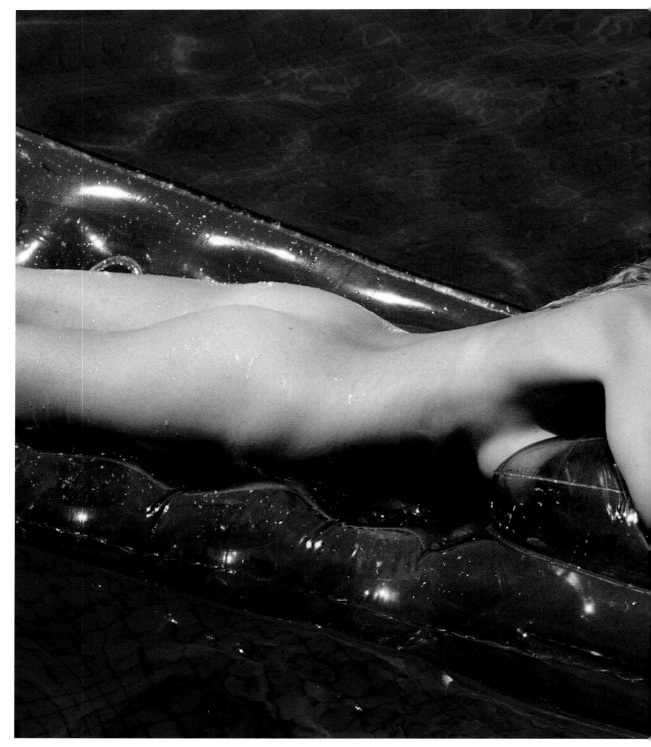

Floating naked, hot sun on bare flesh, a little playful flirting,

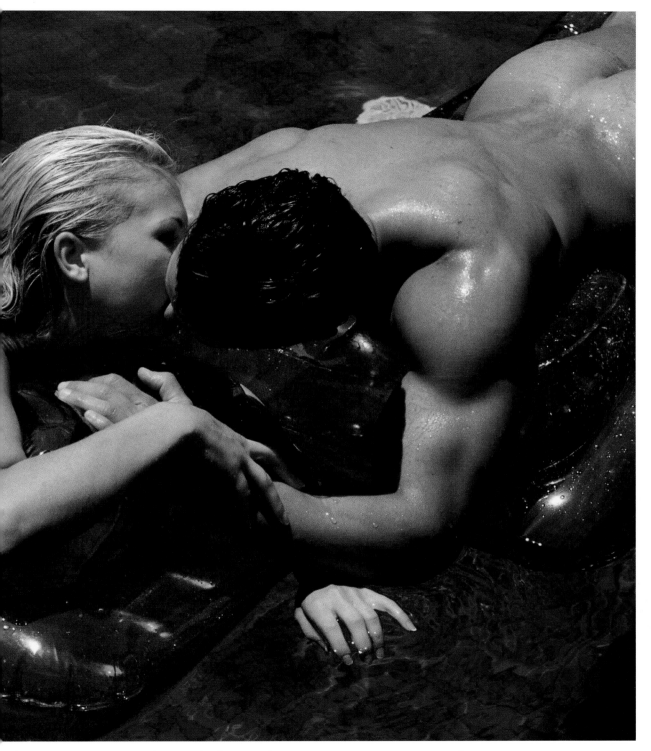

the cool water beneath... change location to change sensation.

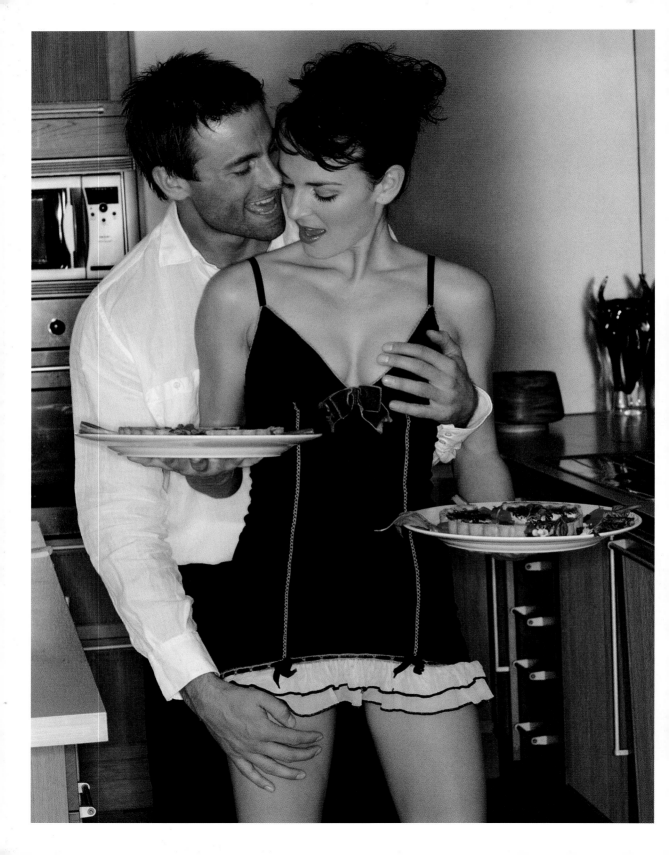

7:10 pm

Your guests are due in 20 minutes, so this quickie had better be quick! To speed things up, grab his buttock cheeks. Big, tempting, orbs of flesh—his bottom tends to be admired in jeans but ignored during sex play. Which is why he'll love it if you move your hands in large circles, massaging and maintaining firm pressure so you indirectly stimulate the anal area. Your grand finale? Reach down to cradle his testicles, pulling them slightly down and away from his body.

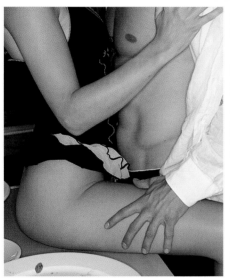

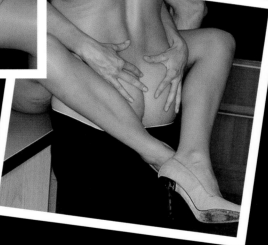

HOME

lustylocation

oh!
oh!
oh!

orgasmoh!meter

riskfactor

she's half-dressed and hurriedly putting the finishing touches on the food; he decides he'd like to add a few touches himself.

naughty stuff...

I'm not turning weird on you and suggesting he buys a flashy gold chain and unbuttons his shirt, while you squeeze into too-tight Lycra, to head hand-in-hand to the local swingers' club. But I do suggest you **explore some new sexual territories**—ones that are perhaps slightly iffier than you're used to. Sweet, snuggly couple sex is affectionate and bonding, but it's the **slightly risqué, darker** variety that tends to put a wicked gleam back into a tired, been-there-done-that-six-billion-times long-term liaison. So **push yourselves out of your comfort zones** and give one of the following a whirl. **Don't think about it too much**—just do it! The worst scenario is you laugh (great) or don't enjoy it (not ideal, but hardly a trauma). The thing is, just by trying, you've instantly made yourself sexier to your partner and **added much-needed va-va-voom.**

1 spanking

You get spanked when you've been naughty—probably one reason why we often associate pain with pleasure. The pleasure came first, the pain is our punishment for it, so the two get linked in our minds. Spanking works two ways: it's a psychological turn-on because it's "wrong" to hit someone, plus spanking our fleshy bits brings the blood to the surface of the skin, making it supersensitive. The trick to expert spanking is striking the right balance: it has to be sharp enough to shock, but not hard enough to actually cause pain. Wait until your partner is excited before attempting it, because our pain receptors are dulled when aroused. The more turned on they are, the more they can take. Use your hand, the back of a hairbrush, or visit a good sex shop or website (there are loads of bondage and discipline specialists) and invest in a soft whip or paddle.

...and why you should try it

2
tie-up games

Bondage (the scary word for tying each other up) works us into an erotic lather because it's a power game. You're either submissive or dominant. Most of us love being submissive, because psychologically we get to surrender all the guilt, hang-ups, and inhibitions that sully our sexual freedom. We're forced to do things we wouldn't dream of ourselves (ahem) and if we turn out to be naturals at it or like it (a lot), well, it's not really our fault, is it?

If you're the dominant one, you're the boss of the bedroom, which brings its own special treats. Everyone knows power corrupts, and even the nicest of us feel a sexy thrill at the political incorrectness of ordering our partner around.

Use braided nylon, soft rope (from most sex shops), PVC (vinyl) tape, specially made cuffs, or long socks. Bedposts, chairs, and staircase railings are good places to start. What to do once you've got them at your mercy? Tease with a capital T!

3
roleplay and dress-up

Rich bitch and the poor, groveling hired help; the cruel brothel boss and a manipulative sex worker; dishy doctor and naughty nurse; boss and secretary; Batman and Robin; and Will and Grace if you fancy it… when it comes to roleplay and dress-up scenarios, you're limited only by your imagination. Or a partner who's worried about looking "silly." Lure them in by providing a traditionally sexy, extremely flattering outfit the first time. Once they've been initiated into the playfulness of dress-up, you can suggest more adventurous character-led outfits.

Dressing up is extremely healthy for relationships because it makes us see our partners differently. Regular contact and familiarity stops us from really "seeing" each other. Dressed in something out of the ordinary, we're forced to look afresh (and hopefully rejoice in what we see).

4
making movies

Most people have watched porn. Imagine how interesting it would be if the characters on screen were you! Lots of couples enjoy both making and watching movies of themselves. You get to see what the two of you really do in bed and, if filmed flatteringly, it can work wonders for a wobbly body image.
• Look your best: Apply fake tan, make-up, and powder to your faces (yes, it works on him too) and a slick of oil to your bodies.
• Mount the camera from above, for flattering angles. Ideally, the lights would be "warm," and would shine from below.
• Overexaggerate everything: If you're using lube, pour a puddle from a height, warm it between your palms, looking first at his penis, then his eyes, then at the camera, letting all know exactly what's going to happen. And talking dirty on film is *de rigueur*.
• I do strongly recommend the female gets to keep the video. Paranoid? Maybe. But invariably it's the female's reputation that is damaged if it falls into the wrong hands.

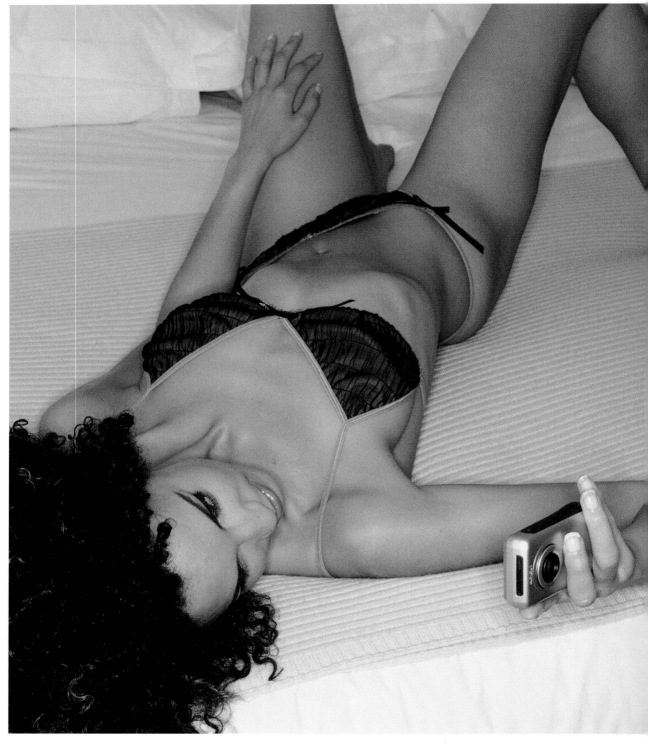

"I love the way you taste," "I want you in my mouth"—simple

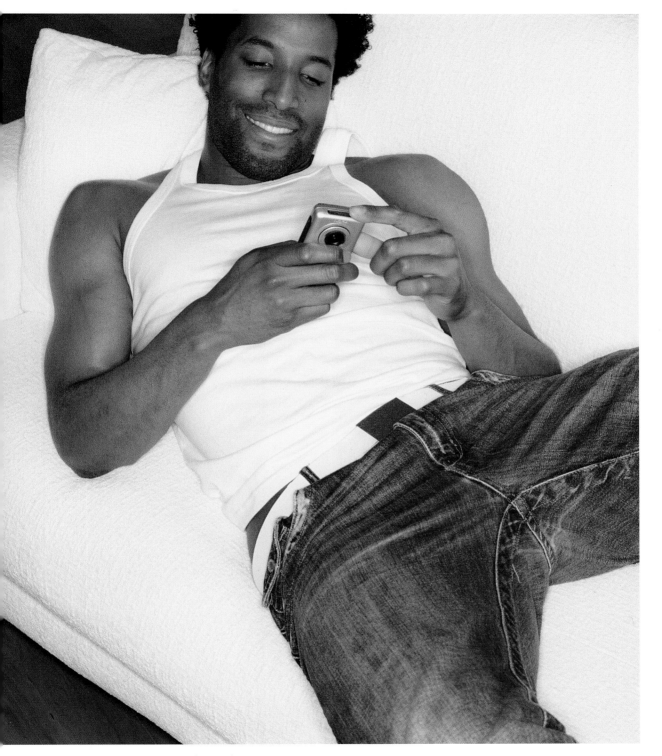

entences pack punch when part of an unexpected sex text.

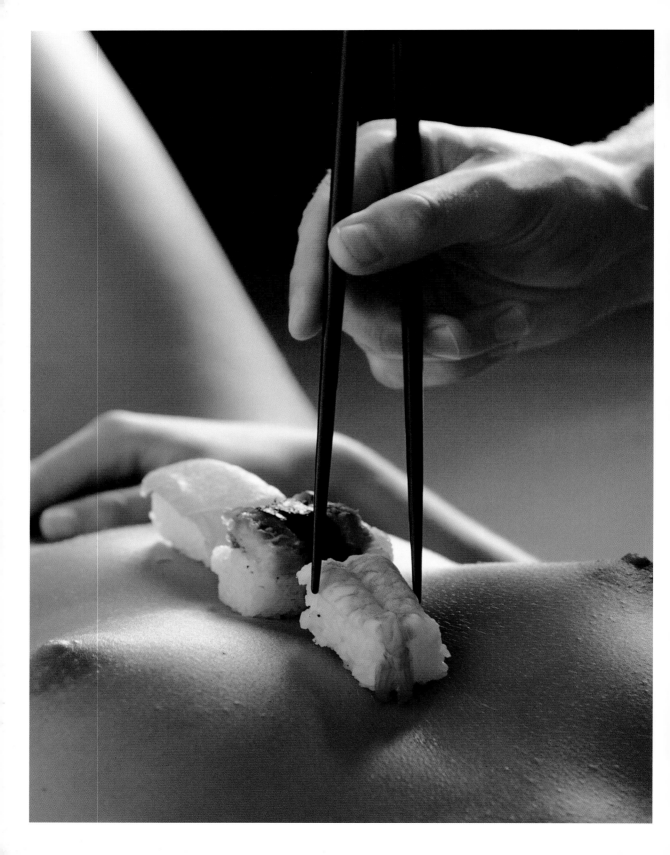

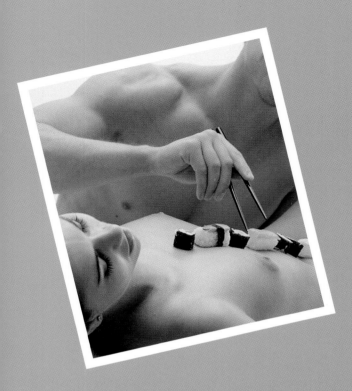

Food and sex—two of life's greatest pleasures. Add a frisky bottle of wine and lots of luxury chocolate and you've landed in most people's idea of hedonist heaven. Kim Basinger revived the "lewd food" concept quite spectacularly in *Nine and a Half Weeks*, but zoologists suspect lovers sharing, feeding, and smearing food on and in each other started around the time the first woolly mammoth got dropped onto hot coals. Food titillates our sense of smell and tickles the taste buds. The right types and textures also feel fantastic on bare skin—licking off anything creamy, fluffy, cold, or gooey stimulates all our senses, providing an extraordinarily erotic treat. Besides, the food/sex combo is incredibly time-efficient because it satisfies two needs at once! Steer clear of hot, spicy, or acidic foods and your kitchen suddenly becomes the sexiest room in the house!

DINNER

lustylocation

oh!
oh!
oh!

orgasmoh!**meter**

riskfactor

You've gotta eat, right? So what's stopping you from eating dinner off each other's naked flesh and satisfying two cravings at once?

9:10 pm

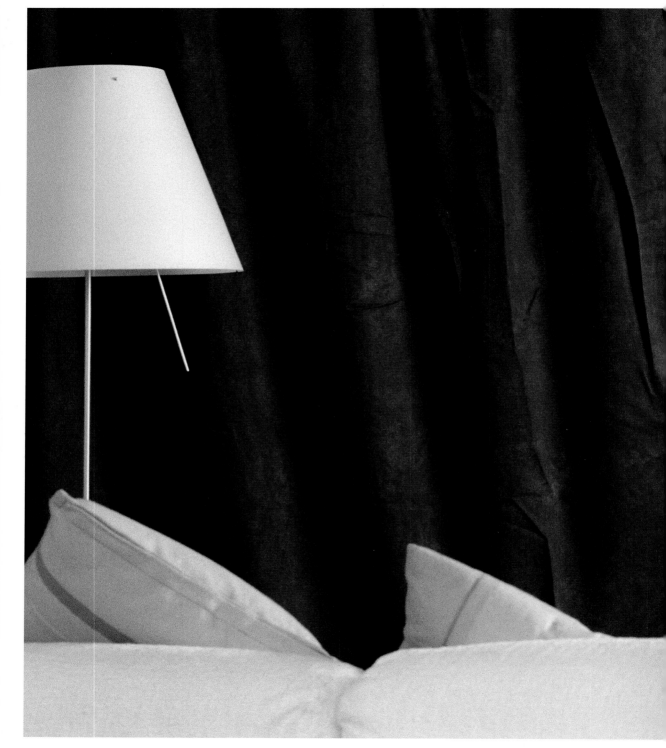

Roleplaying a clandestine affair, you slip behind heavy drapes,

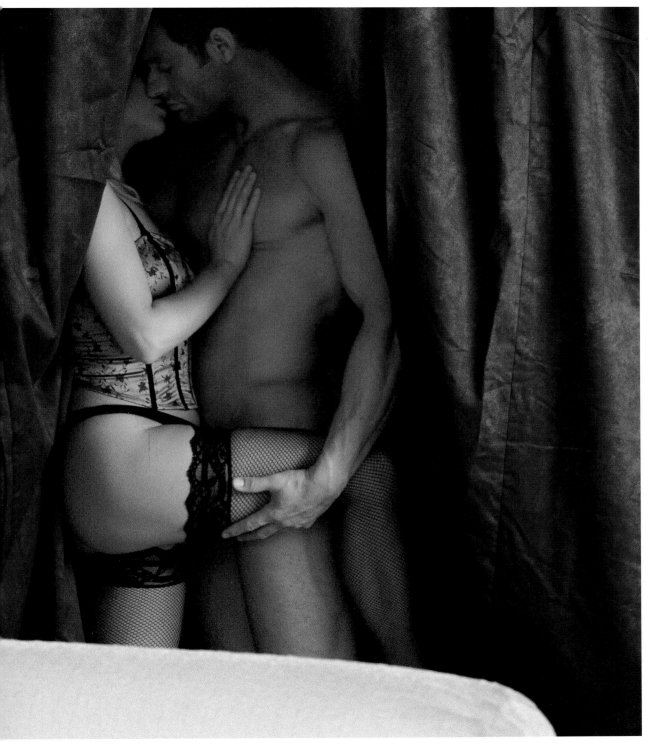

loins aching and hearts pounding for fear of being discovered.

Lust + Love = Happy couple

For quick, connected sex that satisfies body, mind, and soul, keep the following in mind:

KISS

Quick sex doesn't have to be soulless sex—if you half expect your partner to leave a few crisp bills on the nightstand, they're not quite grasping the point. Unless it's deliberately designed to be anonymous, there's no reason why you can't stay connected during the naughtiest, speediest sex encounter. The simplest way to introduce softer emotion to a raw fast fix (without destroying the mood) is to kiss and make eye contact.

KEEP GOING IF YOU CAN

You meant it to be a quickie—you were both trying to lessen the pile of paperwork/ironing/filing that's been haunting you for days. But if somewhere around the five-minute mark, your priorities shift (quite rightly) in favor of longer sex and shorter should-do-the-chores time, go with it. If there's opportunity and energy for something more, let it happen. Rigidly sticking to a time limit because you said you would turns sex back into something with rules attached.

KEEP WATCH

If you're giving it your best shot to ignite a lazy libido but none of the suggestions seem to be working, you might want to seek further help. There's a difference between having a low libido (you don't feel like or focus on sex) and being low-sensation. Low-sensation people feel like sex, but when they have it, they don't feel much. It usually affects women, and there are usually physiological reasons why they experience reduced sensitivity in their nipples, clitoris, or vagina. Pelvic surgery, hormonal changes, stress, depression, medication—all can cause it. A gynecologist or a sex therapist can fix it. Sex therapists can also help shift any psychological blocks that could be stopping you from realizing your full sexual potential. To find a qualified, reputable therapist, visit www.aasect.org (a professional organization with an extensive relationship referral service) or www.sexologist.com (American Board of Sexology, which trains counselors and provides a list of accredited therapists in the US).

KEEP CUDDLING

Yes, you're busy. That's why I've spent the whole book telling you how to maximize sex time. But happy couples need more than just sex to stay content. The same principles you've learned about quickie sex sessions apply to love, too. If you're watching TV, sit together rather than apart. If you feel suffocated snuggled up, connect through just one body part (feet or thighs touching). Put a hand on the small of their back as you pass to grab something. Make it a kiss that connects instead of an air-kiss. Little touches, caresses, and kindnesses go a long way toward keeping the longing as part of the equation.

Quick sex can kick-start a flagging libido, providing an intense shock to the system. She might not always orgasm, but it's great for keeping your sexual systems well-oiled and running smoothly.

KEEP SAFE

I'm encouraging you to push out of your comfort zones, but am also imploring you to be sensible about it. I'm not just wagging a stern finger about the "don't get arrested" stuff, I'm also talking about sexual health when trying things like anal sex. Pay heed to all the warnings, use condoms, and don't try anything that involves trust (tie-up games, etc.) unless you can answer "Yes. Absolutely and totally" within a heartbeat of me asking if you do trust implicitly.

quickie sexcapades

1

"Without any warning at all, she pulled me into the changing room with her, unzipped my pants, and took my penis in her mouth. I could hear the sales clerk come in and tell everyone she was there to help if anyone needed different sizes, and I panicked. There was only a thin curtain separating us, but my girlfriend didn't miss a beat. She fellated me all the way through to orgasm and hid with me until I could make a getaway."

2

"We were at a friend's party and she took me by the hand and led me into a vacant room, then lifted her dress to show me "a surprise." She'd had all her pubic hair waxed off. It meant I could see everything—the outline of the lips, her clitoris protruding, a slick of wetness. We lasted about an hour, then had to go home."

4

"We were walking home from the bar, well lubricated in all senses, when we passed a house that had an open garage—with no car in it. It was set back enough from the road but still risky, since the owner could have driven up at any second. He pushed me against a wall, got down on his knees, pushed my panties to the side, and gave me the best oral I've ever had. Usually, it takes me ages to come, but then I came in about three minutes."

"She'd stand with her hands on a full-length mirror, then ask me to take her doggy style. I felt like I was starring in my own porn movie."

3

"We were getting ready for a dinner party, and I was in the middle of making appetizers. He came up behind me and started kissing my neck, and suddenly I thought, "Forget the guests. I want him now." I reached behind me to push everything off the bench so I could climb on the counter, and most of my hard work ended up on the floor. I'm normally quite an anal person and hell-bent on impressing everyone, but in that instant, I gave in to impulse, and screw the consequences. It turned out to be not just the best sex ever, but the best dinner party. We confessed what happened to the appetizers, and we all ended up drinking too much and swapping embarrassing sex stories. It was incredibly liberating and life-changing. Now I am more in touch with my primitive instincts and a lot more relaxed in general."

5

"We were perched on a rock and I could feel the rough, uneven surface scratching me each time he thrust. It was freezing and my panties got caught around my feet so I couldn't open my legs properly. But it was bruising, nasty sex and I loved it. People use the term "overcome with lust" but I've never felt such an urgent need. Absolutely nothing was going to stop us from doing it right there, right then."

6

"We were crammed at the back of an elevator packed with people, but all were dutifully looking ahead, minding their own business. He put his hand up the back of my dress, and started rubbing my clitoris through my knickers, then pushed them aside and put his fingers inside me. The thrill of being so explicit and intimate in a confined space packed with strangers was the biggest turn-on I've ever had. I still use it to masturbate to."

7

Index

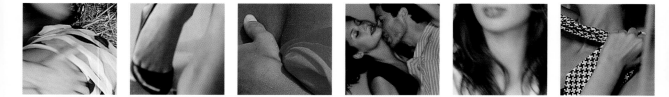

Acknowledgments

It's always risky writing acknowledgments for a book about sex. While some people love getting a mention, dragging the book out at dinner parties and gleefully pointing to their name, other people would rather their contribution be kept private, thank you very much. To those shyer souls, who offered personal inspiration but don't particularly want the world to know how much they enjoy sex in their neighbor's backyard or in the boss's chair, thanks so much for your input.

As for public acknowledgments, I have to thank all the usual suspects: everyone at Dorling Kindersley, worldwide, who works so hard to make my books a success. In the UK office, special thanks to the ever-lovely Corinne Roberts, Deborah Wright, Serena Stent, Hermione Ireland, Liz Statham, Catherine Bell, Adèle Hayward, Nicola Rodway, and my editor, the patient, unflappable Salima Hirani. In the US office, Bill Barry (I'm still gutted you left), Carl Raymond, Therese Burke, Tom Korman, Cathy Sears (who's left her family at DK to look after her own), and Rachel Kempster (returned to us—hurrah!); also to Chris Houston and Loraine Taylor in Canada.

Enormous thanks, as always, to the talented team at XAB—Nigel Wright and Bev Speight—you are not only brilliant designers but fabulous friends. Thanks, daily, to my family—they feel closer every year, even though I live so far away. And never-ending gratitude to my wonderful agent and friend Vicki McIvor, not just for her constant support and love but for choosing me as godmother for the oh-so-precious and adored Lara, her new baby daughter.

DK would like to thank Alyson Lacewing for proofreading and Ted Kinsey for design assistance.

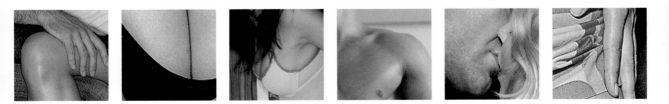

Grab it—and each other—whenever you can. There's nothing like a regular bit of slap-and-tickle to put a wicked twinkle in the eye!

LONDON, NEW YORK, MUNICH,
MELBOURNE, DELHI

Design XAB Design
Senior Editor Salima Hirani
Senior Art Editor Nicola Rodway
Editor Elizabeth Watson
Managing Editor Adèle Hayward
Managing Art Editor Karla Jennings
DTP Designer Julian Dams
Production Controller Sarah Sherlock
Art Director Peter Luff
Publishing Director Corinne Roberts

First American Edition, 2006

Published in the United States by
DK Publishing, Inc., 375 Hudson Street,
New York, NY 10014

06 07 08 09 10   10 9 8 7 6 5 4 3 2 1

Copyright © 2005 Dorling Kindersley Limited
Text copyright © 2005 Tracey Cox

A Cataloging-in-Publication record for this book
is available from the Library of Congress.

ISBN 0-7566-1881-9

DK books are available at special discounts for
bulk purchases for sales promotions, premiums,
fund-raising, or educational use. For details,
contact: DK Publishing Special Markets,
375 Hudson Street, New York, NY 10014 or
SpecialSales@dk.com

Reproduced by GRB, Italy
Cover reproduction by Colourscan, Singapore
Printed and bound by Tien Wah Press, Singapore

The author and publisher would like to urge
readers to remember that the law takes a dim
view of people exposing themselves in public
or offending others—always be discreet (and
avoid getting arrested!).

Discover more at **www.dk.com**

Contents

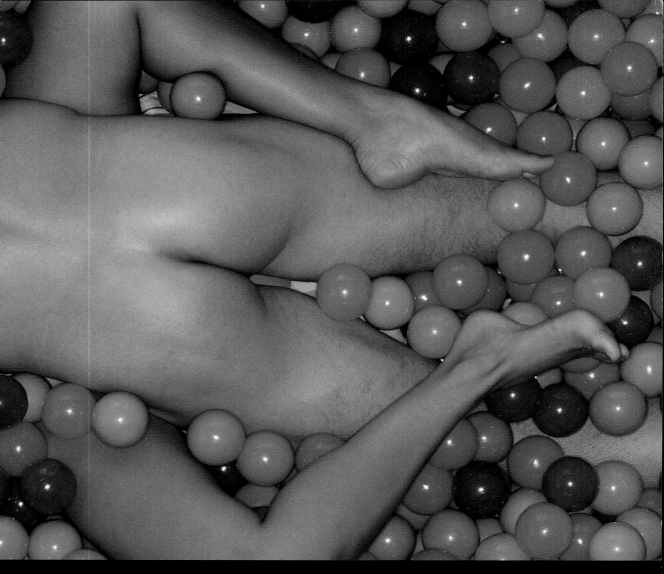

Quickies
tracey cox

photographs by john davis